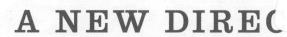
A NEW DIREC

A COGNITIVE-BEHAVIORAL THERAPY PROGRAM

MW00807511

Preparing for Release

SECOND EDITION

WORKBOOK

Minnesota Department of Corrections and Hazelden Publishing

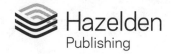

Hazelden
Publishing

Hazelden Publishing
Center City, Minnesota 55012
hazelden.org/bookstore

ISBN: 978-1-61649-787-3

Editor's notes

Some of the quotes in this workbook are from past program participants who appear
in A New Direction videos. Other quotes in this workbook are composites, which were
created to represent the experiences of past program participants.

This publication is not intended as a substitute for the advice of health care professionals.

Readers should be aware that websites listed in this work may have changed or
disappeared between when this work was written and when it is read.

Alcoholics Anonymous and AA are registered trademarks of Alcoholics Anonymous
World Services, Inc.

The *Preparing for Release* workbook, formerly titled *Release & Reintegration
Preparation,* is part of *A New Direction: A Cognitive-Behavioral Therapy Program,*
which was formerly titled *A New Direction: A Cognitive-Behavioral Treatment
Curriculum.*

Cover design: Tom Heffron

Contents

Duplicating this page is illegal. Do not copy this material without written permission from the publisher.

iii

Acknowledgments

Thanks to all who contributed to the second edition of this program:

Paul Schnell
Commissioner, Minnesota Department of Corrections

Joseph Jaksha
Publisher, Hazelden Publishing

Dianne Seger
Associate Director of Behavioral Health, Minnesota Department of Corrections

MINNESOTA DEPARTMENT OF CORRECTIONS
TREATMENT PROGRAMS

Atlantis	Stillwater Correctional Facility
Changing P.A.T.H.S.	Shakopee Correctional Facility
Compass (Challenge Incarceration Program)	Shakopee Correctional Facility
New Dimensions	Faribault Correctional Facility
Paradigm	Moose Lake Correctional Facility
Portages (Challenge Incarceration Program)	Togo Correctional Facility
Positive Changes (Challenge Incarceration Program)	Willow River Correctional Facility
RESHAPE	St. Cloud Correctional Facility
RIVERS	St. Cloud Correctional Facility
Serenity West	Lino Lakes Correctional Facility
Sex Offender Treatment Program (SOTP)	Lino Lakes Correctional Facility
TRIAD	Lino Lakes Correctional Facility

MINNESOTA DEPARTMENT OF CORRECTIONS
A NEW DIRECTION REVISION COMMITTEE

Emily Ahl, Corrections Program Director	RESHAPE, St. Cloud
Michael Froemke, Corrections Program Director	Positive Changes, Willow River
Marina Fuhrman, Corrections Program Director	Atlantis, Stillwater
Tabitha Jeffries, Corrections Program Director	New Dimensions, Faribault
Colleen Kietzer, Corrections Program Director	TRIAD, Lino Lakes
Janel Lindgren, Corrections Program Director	TRIAD, Lino Lakes

Holly Mans, Corrections Program Director . . . . TRIAD, Lino Lakes

Erica Meier, Corrections Program Director . . . . New Dimensions, Faribault

Megan Moeller, Corrections Program Director . . . . Central Office, St. Paul

Jolene Rebertus, Director, Health Services
   Release Planning . . . . Central Office, St. Paul

Tami Thon, Corrections Program Director . . . . TRIAD, Lino Lakes

Rhonda Vahle, Psychological Services Director . . . . TRIAD, Lino Lakes

Angela Vatalaro, Corrections Program Director . . . . Paradigm, Moose Lake

HAZELDEN PUBLISHING

Writers: Cynthia Orange, Jessica Orange

Editors: Anita Dincesen, Abby Karels, Drew Siqveland, Sue Thomas

Editorial Project Managers: Jean Cook, April Ebb, Don Freeman

Copyeditor: Sally Heuer

Proofreaders: Catherine Broberg, Monica Dwyer Frischkorn

Art Director: Terri Kinne

Typesetters: Trina Christensen, Terri Kinne, Nancy Whittlesey

Illustrator: Patrice Barton

Video Production Manager: Wes Thomsen

Video Production: Blue Moon Productions

Training Manager: Lily Kreitinger

Marketing Manager: Alice Cunningham

Administrative Assistant: Nicole Arends

SPECIAL THANKS

- All who contributed to the development of the first edition of A New Direction

- The facility administration, staff, and offenders of the Minnesota Correctional Facility–Lino Lakes and the Minnesota Correctional Facility–Stillwater for their invaluable support

- The treatment participants from the Minnesota Correctional Facility–Lino Lakes and the Minnesota Correctional Facility–Stillwater for their diligent feedback on the workbooks

- The alumni of the treatment programs at the Minnesota Correctional Facility– Lino Lakes and the Minnesota Correctional Facility–Stillwater for their inspiring stories of recovery

Introduction

By the end of this chapter, you will be able to	• identify individual areas of life to focus on for reentry
	• identify factors that reduce the risk of relapse
	• describe the importance of setting SMART goals

The closer we get to our release date, the more we realize how much our lives are about to change. Everything might seem different upon release because *we* are different now. We have learned how important it is to stay crime free and abstinent from alcohol and other drugs. We've learned essential skills for how to remain crime free and abstinent, which is one of the ways we are different. These skills are important to keep in mind as we prepare for release. We can use what we've learned to help ourselves do things differently.

Release can be a positive experience. It's common to have fears, and it's okay to be afraid. We hope this workbook will help ease these fears. We aren't the only thing that will be different. A lot of things have changed since we were incarcerated. Being prepared for that will help us to better manage the stress that comes with change. The longer we've been away, the more changes we will likely notice. Some things, such as the old criminal crowd, may not have changed. But we've learned about the dangers of our past behavior and know more about our risks for relapse.

Right now we're living in a world that is guided by rules and structure. There are people who help create structure for us and who make sure that we follow the rules. But that will change after we're released. We will have more time to ourselves and less supervision. We are responsible for our own thoughts, behaviors, and actions. That's a big change *and* a big challenge. But we've learned a lot about ourselves, and this workbook provides tools that will help us overcome the challenges we will face.

Before we are released, we need to start thinking about some important parts of our lives. For example, we'll need to decide where to live. We'll also need to find a job. And we'll need to choose who to spend time with and what to do for fun. In deciding all of this, it is normal to have doubts that we'll be able to stay abstinent. This workbook will help us make plans and set specific, realistic goals. *But no matter what, our most important goal is to stay abstinent.*

EXERCISE 1.1	REFLECTION

What are your thoughts and questions right now? Describe three things you are thinking about as you begin this workbook.

1. _____

2. _____

3. _____

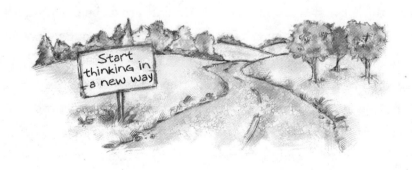

We've learned a lot about ourselves, and this workbook provides tools that will help us overcome the challenges we will face.

Duplicating this page is illegal. Do not copy this material without written permission from the publisher.

Reentry Is Different for Everyone

We all have areas in life that present challenges. There are unique challenges to living under supervision, and there are also unique challenges that come with being released. As we prepare for reentry, it can be helpful to look at the different areas of our lives that might cause problems for us. In fact, there are even tests that can help predict which areas increase the risk of reoffending. There is no one-size-fits-all approach to reentry. Exploring and addressing our problem areas can help each of us to come up with our own individual recovery plan that increases our chances of success. Here are some common high-risk areas:

- criminal history
- school/work
- family/marriage
- friends
- free time

- alcohol and other drugs
- attitudes
- thoughts and emotions
- housing
- finances

EXERCISE 1.2   REFLECTION

1. Review the areas of risk that we just listed. Which areas present the greatest challenges for you?

   _____

   _____

2. Describe why these are challenging areas for you.

   _____

   _____

3. List some helpful ways you can deal with these challenges.

   _____

   _____

Core Beliefs

As we've already learned, we have to look "upstream" to see what *core beliefs* led to our thoughts and decisions, which in turn led to our behavior and actions. If we were to draw how this works, it might look like this:

Event → Core Beliefs → Thoughts → Feelings → Behavior

Remember that core beliefs are the "thoughts behind our thoughts." They are the thoughts we've long accepted as true. Some of these core beliefs are healthy and protect us, but some are not and can lead to distorted thinking that can then lead to unhealthy or criminal behavior. Stopping our use of alcohol and other drugs and stopping our criminal activities does not change the way we think. We have to pay attention to our thoughts, which can then lead us to understand our core beliefs. When we understand our unhealthy core beliefs, we can work to replace them with healthy ones, and that can help us prevent relapse and stay on track with our recovery. The goal is to change our thinking problems before they become behavior problems. Each of us has our own core beliefs that we can work to improve.

Here are some examples of core beliefs:

- **I always fail.** (view of self)

- **I deserve special treatment.** (view of self)

- **My future is hopeful.** (view of self)

- **It's me versus authority.** (view of other people)

- **You can't trust people.** (view of other people)

- **People will help if I ask for help.** (view of other people)

- **The system is always stacked against me.** (view of the world)

- **It's a dog-eat-dog world.** (view of the world)

- **The world rewards people who work hard.** (view of the world)

1. Which core beliefs present the greatest challenges for you?

   _____

   _____

2. Describe why these might be challenging for you after release.

   _____

   _____

3. List some ways you can change these core beliefs.

   _____

   _____

Thinking Distortions

Thinking distortions are inaccurate, slanted, or one-sided ways that people look at themselves, other people, and the world. Thinking distortions lead to thoughts and beliefs that may sound good on the surface or have some slight truth to them. But thinking distortions mix up reality so our thinking becomes faulty. Distortions in how we think can lead to other distorted thoughts, to distorted behaviors (criminality, irresponsibility, addiction), and to distressing emotions (anxiety, rage, depression). Each of us has our own thinking distortions that we can recognize and try to challenge.

> *Thinking distortions are inaccurate, slanted, or one-sided ways that people look at themselves, other people, and the world.*

Duplicating this page is illegal. Do not copy this material without written permission from the publisher.

INTRODUCTION • **5**

Here are some of the major thinking distortions used by people who commit crimes or have an addiction:

- **extreme thinking** (all-or-nothing thinking), when we view everything as one extreme or another

- **overgeneralization** ("always" or "never" thinking), when we think that if something happened once or twice, it must always be true

- **personalization** (making everything about us), when we only see things from our point of view and think everything that happens around us is all about us

- **magnification and minimization** (making something seem greater or smaller than it really is), when we take an event out of context and blow it out of proportion, or we downplay its impact or significance

- **jumping to conclusions** (assuming something without getting all the facts), when we think we know something and make snap decisions with no evidence

- **selective focus** (looking at only one small piece of what happened), when we focus only on certain parts of a story or situation

- **concrete thinking** (stubborn, "I know what's right" thinking), when we focus on details but don't understand the message behind them

- **actor versus observer** (thinking we are never at fault or responsible for our behavior), when we believe situations just happen to us and we don't take responsibility for our actions

- **closed thinking** (no one can tell us differently), when we don't listen or trust new information

- **emotional reasoning** (making conclusions based on our feelings), when we believe that our feelings are facts

Thinking Distortions
- extreme thinking
- overgeneralization
- personalization
- magnification and minimization
- jumping to conclusions
- selective focus
- concrete thinking
- actor versus observer
- closed thinking
- emotional reasoning

1. Which thinking distortions present the greatest challenges for you?

   _____

2. Describe why these might be challenging for you after release.

   _____

   _____

   _____

3. List some ways you can change or challenge these thinking distortions.

   _____

   _____

   _____

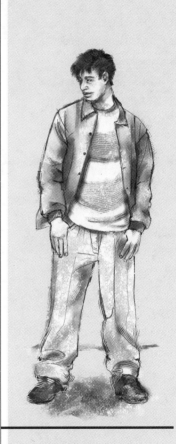

Criminal and Addictive Thinking Patterns

A person who has committed crimes and who has a substance use disorder has developed both criminal and addictive thinking patterns. These thinking patterns aren't all the thoughts we have, but they do dominate our thinking. This can lead to serious trouble. Although people who commit a crime may think about it for a long time without acting on these thoughts, when they do actually commit the crime, they usually do it on the spur of the moment. Addictive thinking patterns fool us into thinking it's okay to use alcohol and other drugs as much as we want, as often as we want, and to do whatever we need to do to get them. Each of us has our own criminal and addictive thinking patterns that we can work to change.

Each of us has our own criminal and addictive thinking patterns that we can work to change.

Basic criminal and addictive thinking patterns are listed here:

- **"victim" or "self-pity" stance,** when we make excuses, point fingers at others, and claim that we were the ones who were wronged

- **"good person" stance,** when we consider ourselves to be a good person, no matter what we do or how we act

- **"unique person" stance,** when we see ourselves as different or special

- **fear of exposure,** when we may act fearless, but inside we are consumed with fear

- **lack of time perspective,** when we tend to live only in the present or in the near future

- **selective effort,** when we do almost anything to avoid responsible effort

- **use of power or deceit to control,** when we use power to manipulate, intimidate, humiliate, or dominate others or when we lie, cheat, steal, and beg to get what we want

- **seek excitement or pleasure first,** when we seek excitement first, which keeps us from responsible behavior, or when we seek the pleasure of getting high without thinking about the consequences

- **"ownership" stance,** when we have a distorted view of which rights and property are ours and which belong to others

Addictive thinking patterns fool us into thinking it's okay to use alcohol and other drugs as much as we want, as often as we want, and to do whatever we need to do to get them.

Criminal and Addictive Thinking Patterns

- "victim" or "self-pity" stance
- "good person" stance
- "unique person" stance
- fear of exposure
- lack of time perspective
- selective effort
- use of power or deceit to control
- seek excitement or pleasure first
- "ownership" stance

1. Which criminal and addictive thinking patterns present the greatest challenges for you?

_____

2. Describe why these might be challenging for you after release.

_____

_____

_____

3. List some ways you can change these criminal and addictive thinking patterns.

_____

_____

Tactics

Criminal and addictive tactics can be divided into three categories: avoidance strategies, diversion strategies, and aggression strategies. We use *avoidance strategies* to escape responsibility, to keep a low profile so we won't have to put out effort or be exposed, and to manipulate others to get what we want. We use *diversion strategies* to confuse others, to direct attention away from ourselves or from important issues, and to avoid exposure by keeping those around us distracted and focused on other things. We use *aggression strategies* to attack, intimidate, and undermine the efforts of others.

When we behave responsibly, we use responsible tactics to accomplish something helpful and worthwhile for ourselves, our families, or our communities. When we behave irresponsibly, we use irresponsible tactics to get something for ourselves without earning it. We hide our true motives to take advantage of others and avoid responsibility. Each of us has our own tactics that we can work to change. The following table lists common criminal and addictive tactics.

Criminal and Addictive Tactics

1. avoidance strategies

2. diversion strategies

3. aggression strategies

Common Criminal and Addictive Tactics

Avoidance Strategies	Diversion Strategies	Aggression Strategies
Lying by omission	Pointing out the faults of others	Arguing
Being deliberately vague	Magnifying (exaggerating significance)	Using threatening words or behaviors (veiled or direct)
Staying silent to avoid notice	Deliberately trying to confuse	Raging
False compliance (pretending to say or do the "right" thing)	Quibbling over words	Using sarcasm and teasing
Playing dumb	Introducing irrelevant issues	Splitting staff
Using selective memory and attention	Discussing smokescreen issues	Creating chaos
Minimizing (trivializing)	Using self-shaming to avoid responsibility	Attention seeking

EXERCISE 1.6   **REFLECTION**

1. Which criminal and addictive tactics present the greatest challenges for you?

   _____

2. Describe why these might be challenging for you after release.

   _____

   _____

   _____

3. List some ways you can change these tactics.

   _____

   _____

Based on what you have read so far in this chapter, fill in the blanks to complete these statements.

1. Core beliefs are the "_____ behind our thoughts."

2. _____ _____ are inaccurate, slanted, or one-sided ways that people look at themselves, others, and the world.

3. _____ _____ _____ fool us into thinking it's okay to use alcohol and other drugs as much as we want, as often as we want, and to do whatever we need to do to get them.

4. Criminal and addictive tactics can be divided into three categories: _____ strategies, _____ strategies, and _____ strategies.

Factors That Reduce the Risk of Relapse

Most of us leave the criminal justice system determined to stay out of it forever. But we know that it takes hard work to stay abstinent and crime free. We need to know what to look out for when we get released—the things that could put us at risk for relapse. And the best place to start is with our thinking.

Healthy Thinking Patterns

Our thinking is like a map—a map our minds use to get around. When we're somewhere new, not just any old map will do; we need a good map. Our mental map tells us about what's going on. Without it, we are lost. But our map can also mislead us. Maps become old. As our lives change and we grow older, our map needs to change too. If it doesn't change, it becomes faulty. When this happens, we interpret situations in ways that lead to trouble. We've learned to accept responsibility for our thoughts, feelings, and actions, and not to use power or lies to control or humiliate others.

We need to know what to look out for when we get released—the things that could put us at risk for relapse. And the best place to start is with our thinking.

Duplicating this page is illegal. Do not copy this material without written permission from the publisher.

INTRODUCTION • 11

The good news is, we're in charge of our own mental map. We've learned about core beliefs, thinking distortions, and criminal and addictive thinking patterns and tactics. We can use that knowledge to improve our thinking. We can change our core beliefs so that they are healthier and support our recovery. We can learn how to erase the faulty parts of our mental map and instead create a new, more effective map that will help us to reach our goals.

Relapse Prevention

One of our biggest challenges is to prevent *relapse*. Relapse is a process of returning to substance use or criminal behavior after a period of not using and not being involved in a criminal lifestyle. Our situations are unique because we have criminal records. When we relapse, we might end up right back where we are now. Worse yet, we could end up dead.

Relapse starts long before we take a drink, use a drug, or commit a crime. Stress, poor coping skills, and poor decision-making skills can all cause us to make seemingly unimportant decisions that bring us closer and closer to a high-risk situation. And risky situations can lead us to relapse. Relapse is always possible—it doesn't matter how long we've been sober or crime free.

Relapses are not caused by a lack of willpower or because something is wrong with our character. They are caused by unhealthy coping skills that we use to manage our addiction and criminal behavior. Healthy skills, attitudes, and information can help us prevent relapse or stop relapses when they happen. We just need to practice the healthy skills.

We may not relapse with our original drug or criminal behavior, and our substance use or criminal behavior may not be as severe as it once was. Nevertheless, it is important to recognize a relapse. The link is strong between our criminal and our addictive behaviors. If we do something unlawful, there's a better chance we'll start using substances again and vice versa. That's why relapse prevention is so important after we get released.

One of the key skills to learn in recovery is how to *prevent* a relapse from both substance use and criminal activity. And we also need to learn how to *stop* our substance use or criminal activity if we do relapse. If we have relapse prevention skills, we increase our chances of abstinence after release. And if we stay abstinent after our release, we increase our chances at successful long-term recovery. Helpful relapse prevention skills include

- maintaining a balanced lifestyle
- identifying external and internal triggers
- coping with cravings
- avoiding or coping with high-risk situations
- developing a support network
- creating a relapse prevention plan
- creating an emergency plan for relapse or a major setback in life

EXERCISE 1.8	REFLECTION

1. List some ways that you can continue to improve your thinking patterns after release.

   _____

   _____

2. List effective relapse prevention skills that can help you after release.

   _____

   _____

If we have relapse prevention skills, we increase our chances of abstinence after release. And if we stay abstinent after our release, we increase our chances at successful long-term recovery.

We've been talking about what we can do internally, such as thinking in healthier ways and practicing our relapse prevention skills. Now we'll look at some positive ways to put our skills into practice. There are things we can do to reduce our risk of relapse—practicing them will help us to stay focused on our recovery after release.

Healthy Socialization

Socialization is about us and our relationships with other people. It's also about living and behaving in a way that is acceptable to society. We need a good relationship with ourselves if we want healthy relationships with others. If we understand the difference between healthy and unhealthy relationships, we can build and maintain relationships that support our recovery. This is important as we reenter our communities and have more freedom around our interactions with others.

Our personal and family histories can be a good place to start. Both of them affected the way we developed, and knowing that helps us understand where we may need to make some changes. Positive changes can support our goals after release. Here are some examples of helpful ways to improve our socialization:

- Identify trustworthy relationships.
- Build healthy relationships.
- Choose a therapist.
- Find a sponsor or mentor.
- Attend a recovery support group.
- Seek spiritual support.
- Build a positive relationship with a parole and/or probation officer.

It's crucial to remember that the goal in human relationships is *interdependence*. We need other healthy people in our lives in order to survive and thrive. And they need us too.

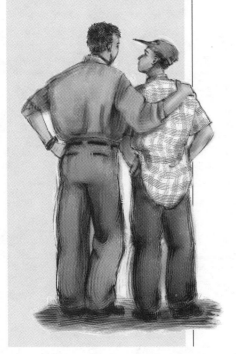

We need a good relationship with ourselves if we want healthy relationships with others.

Sober Fun

It's important to have fun with others. But we need to be thoughtful about what activities we choose to do with friends and family. Many of us got into the habit of thinking that having fun involved crime and the use of alcohol and other drugs. We know now that thinking that way will put our recovery at risk. There are sober activities we can have fun doing instead, as long as these activities are not associated with substance use or criminal behavior.

By enjoying sober activities, we can find new hobbies—things we regularly do that help maintain our recovery. Here are some examples of hobbies that can help us stay abstinent and support long-term recovery, as long as we do not associate them with substance use or criminal behavior:

- biking
- reading
- drawing
- journaling
- gardening
- fishing
- photography
- playing a sport
- working out/exercising
- crafting/building something
- hiking
- playing a musical instrument

| EXERCISE 1.9 | REFLECTION |

1. List some ways to help yourself have healthy socialization after release.

_____

_____

2. List some sober activities you can do to have fun after release.

_____

_____

Duplicating this page is illegal. Do not copy this material without written permission from the publisher.

INTRODUCTION • 15

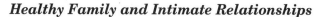

Healthy Family and Intimate Relationships

A *family* is a system, or unit, that is made up of a number of individuals. Some of these people are related by blood, while others are not. Whether we live with them or not, families have the ability to affect and influence us.

In unhealthy families, rules can be confusing, boundaries may not be respected, and secrecy and shame often keep people from talking openly about problems. Family members may not feel valued and may fear doing anything that goes against the "family code." Healthy families, on the other hand, tend to have good communication and a foundation of respect. Family members know what to expect from one another and have rules that are positive and consistent. They trust one another and feel valued. No family is 100 percent healthy or unhealthy; most families are somewhere in between. If our traditional family is not abstinent or supportive of our recovery, we may need to seek out people we consider to be like family who support our recovery.

An intimate and meaningful relationship can happen between couples as well as with friends and family members. Although the word *intimacy* is often associated with sex, intimate relationships don't always have to be sexual. Intimacy means being emotionally connected and close through a variety of activities that are informal, deep, and personal. To be intimate, both people need to be honest and respectful of each other and openly share their thoughts and feelings. Both people should be willing to admit their own faults rather than pointing out the faults of the other person. This requires being open-minded and willing to hear the other person's point of view, as well as compromising when disagreements arise.

Those of us with children also need to remember that our kids need parents. They need time, direction, and attention from us. They need and deserve to be respected as human beings, not as things or possessions. Almost nothing in life is more important than having a positive effect on the lives of our children.

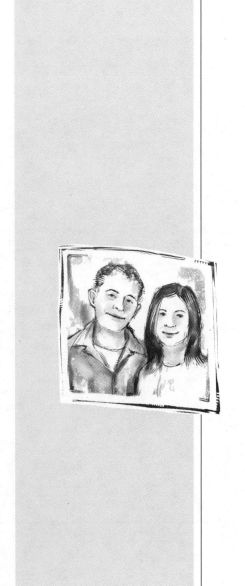

School/Work

Most of us will need to look for a job when we are released, though some of us may choose to go to school instead. Some of us might even work *and* go to school. Preparing for challenges related to work and school can help us reduce the risk of returning to unhealthy behaviors.

Applying for jobs and schooling can be stressful. Our criminal history and past use of alcohol and other drugs can make things even harder. It can be difficult to balance the time we spend on work and education with other parts of our lives, such as time with our families or recovery meetings. We may worry about how much money we'll be making or feel pressure to perform well. We may even need to think about how to handle tension with co-workers or how to stay away from those who use substances at work or at school.

We've learned that thinking about things in advance, such as school or work, allows us to prepare for any stresses that might show up in the future. Being prepared is part of a healthy approach to school and work, which in turn will help us to stay focused on our recovery.

Mental Health

In addition to our criminal history and addiction, some of us also have *co-occurring disorders*—mental health conditions that affect how our brains work. These conditions include depression, anxiety, and bipolar disorder. Co-occurring disorders are serious brain diseases, but fortunately treatment is available. Many people with co-occurring disorders seek help and find the relief they have been looking for all their lives. People can and do recover.

Treating co-occurring disorders at the same time as our criminal and addictive thinking can also help us to stay on the path to recovery. We can seek help with treatment of co-occurring disorders and learn how to overcome common barriers to treatment. Having co-occurring disorders doesn't define who we are. Instead, it means we have symptoms that we need to learn to manage in order to stay healthy.

Treating co-occurring disorders at the same time as our criminal and addictive thinking can also help us to stay on the path to recovery. Having co-occurring disorders doesn't define who we are. Instead, it means we have symptoms that we need to learn to manage in order to stay healthy.

1. What are some things you can do after release to promote healthy relationships for yourself and others?

   _____

   _____

   _____

2. What are some things you can do after release to promote a healthy approach to school and/or work?

   _____

   _____

   _____

3. If you have co-occurring disorders, what are some healthy ways you can manage your mental health after release?

   _____

   _____

   _____

   _____

   _____

   _____

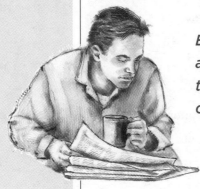

Being prepared is part of a healthy approach to school and work, which in turn will help us to stay focused on our recovery.

Set Goals for Yourself

Setting goals is a great way to make changes. Without changes, how can we expect our lives to be any different after we are released than they were before? If we set specific, healthy, and realistic goals, we can build a future that supports recovery and is free from criminal activity and substance use.

The types of goals we set for ourselves will help us track our progress. One way to increase our chances of success is to be smart about the goals we set for ourselves. And an easy way to remember how to do that is to set "SMART" goals:

- **<u>S</u>pecific:** The more specific a goal is, the easier it is to track progress.

- **<u>M</u>easurable:** Staying on track is easy when we know how to measure success.

- **<u>A</u>chievable:** A successful goal is one that we are able to reach.

- **<u>R</u>elevant:** To be relevant, a goal, and its timing, should be right for us.

- **<u>T</u>ime-bound:** Part of setting a goal is determining when we hope to achieve it.

EXERCISE 1.11   **QUICK REVIEW**

Based on what you just read, fill in the blanks below.

1. Setting _____ is a great way to make changes.

2. SMART goals are

   S _____

   M _____

   A _____

   R _____

   T _____

Goals of This Workbook

By reading the material in this workbook and completing the exercises in it, you can better prepare yourself for release.

The four goals of this *Preparing for Release* workbook are to help you

1. describe a healthy recovery environment that includes supervision and social support
2. identify goals related to employment, finances, and fun
3. explain how health and wellness fit into ongoing recovery efforts
4. develop a recovery plan for after release

Chapter Summary

In this chapter, we learned that we all have our own experience with release. We discussed how to examine our own problem areas and how to address our thinking patterns. We identified some things that increase our risk of relapse, and we thought about ways to help ourselves deal with those things. Finally, we learned what SMART goals are and how they can help us achieve long-term recovery success after release.

SMART Goals

- **S**pecific
- **M**easurable
- **A**chievable
- **R**elevant
- **T**ime-bound

2

Living under Supervision

By the end of this chapter, you will be abie to	• identify personal feelings related to living under supervision
	• describe the roles and expectations associated with living under supervision after release
	• identify ways to build a positive relationship with a supervising authority
	• describe ways to ask for help

Statistics show that after release, many people run the risk of returning to prison. In fact, the first few days or weeks after release pose the greatest risk for people as they return to the community. Preparing for release is an important part of transitioning into a new lifestyle with less supervision. The skills we learn in this workbook will help to better prepare us for that.

Right now, we're used to living under supervision and we know what's expected from us. After release, we'll be in a new environment where expectations will be different. But we'll still need to report regularly to an assigned authority figure. This is usually a parole or probation officer. By learning about how to live under supervision in a new environment after release, we increase our chances of long-term recovery success.

Release Concerns

Even though we are being granted release, our release comes with conditions. Some of us might be required to wear an electronic monitoring device. Some of us may need to follow a curfew. People get released under different conditions, but some general things will be expected of all of us. For example, we will be expected to find a place to live and to find a job or enroll in school. We will be expected to participate in random testing for alcohol and other drugs. And most of us will likely be assigned a parole officer (PO) or other supervising authority who will randomly check in with us, both at work and at home.

Release into the community under supervision involves a much less structured environment than being incarcerated. That means we will have more freedom, but it also means we must take on more responsibility. Our supervising authority is someone who can help us adjust to and manage our freedom. He or she will help us reintegrate, which is an important step toward being free from correctional supervision. The supervising authority assigned to us might be a parole officer, a probation officer, or someone else.

The idea of living under supervision irritates many of us. But we can think about it another way—supervised release is a chance for us to prove that we are focused on long-term recovery, both from criminal behavior and from alcohol and other drugs. It is a chance for us to prove that we are ready for unsupervised release. After all, everyone must deal with some form of supervision, whether from a landlord, employer, teacher, spiritual advisor, or someone else.

Our supervising authority is someone who can help us adjust to and manage our freedom.

1. Describe how you feel about supervised release.

   _____

   _____

2. What are your biggest concerns related to supervised release?

   _____

   _____

3. List some healthy ways you might address those concerns and list other people who might be able to help you.

   _____

   _____

   _____

   _____

   _____

So much of our recovery involves facing our fears. To face our fears, we must first admit that we have them. This isn't an easy thing to do. But we are all afraid of something. Some of us are afraid of relapsing. Some of us are afraid of screwing up and getting into more trouble with the law. And some of us have fears related to living under supervision. This could be because of personal bias.

A bias is a positive or negative judgment that affects our outlook. Our biases affect how we act and interact with others. For example, a positive bias toward our children might lead us to believe they can do no wrong. Or a negative bias toward the police might lead us to believe they want us to screw up.

Bias

A **bias** is a positive or negative judgment that affects our outlook.

1. What are your biases about living under supervision?

2. How do your feelings about supervised release relate to your biases about living under supervision?

3. How are your core beliefs related to your biases about living under supervision?

4. How might changing your thinking help you better manage life under supervision?

Think about an *event* when you experienced a problem while you were being supervised. Consider what your *thoughts* were and the *feelings* that came from those thoughts. Then report what you did (your *behavior*) as a result of those thoughts. Next, try to figure out your *core beliefs* that may have led you to those thoughts. After that, try to imagine *alternative thoughts* and *alternative behaviors* that wouldn't cause problems for you. Finally, what *thinking distortions, thinking patterns,* and *tactics* can you identify when you review your thoughts and behaviors around this particular event? Review the Example Thinking Report on the next page. Then you will complete one on your own on page 26.

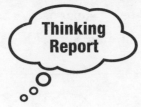

Thinking Report

1. **Event** _A corrections officer came in and searched my cell._

2. **Thoughts** _"Security thinks I'm hiding something. Someone lied and said I have contraband._
   Security wants me to get in trouble."

3. **Feelings** _anger, fear_

4. **Behavior** _I yelled at the officer. I was intentionally uncooperative._

5. **Core Beliefs** _Authority is out to get me. The system is always stacked against me._

6. **Alternative Thoughts** _"Maybe it was my turn to be searched on a random rotation."_

7. **Alternative Behaviors** _When informed about a search, cooperate and calmly ask why._

Thinking Distortions _jumping to conclusions, magnification_

Thinking Patterns _use of power to control; "victim" stance_

Tactics _raging_

Complete a Thinking Report for a problematic event that involved being supervised. Then ask your facilitator for feedback or discuss it with your group.

Thinking Report

1. **Event** _____

_____

2. **Thoughts** _____

_____

3. **Feelings** _____

_____

4. **Behavior** _____

_____

5. **Core Beliefs** _____

_____

6. **Alternative Thoughts** _____

_____

7. **Alternative Behaviors** _____

_____

Thinking Distortions _____

_____

Thinking Patterns _____

_____

Tactics _____

_____

Interacting Positively with Our Supervising Authority

If we have the right attitude and behavior, supervised release can be a positive experience. A supervising authority will play an important role in our lives after release. Because of this, it will be helpful to build a positive relationship with whoever is assigned to work with us. A good place to start is understanding what a positive relationship with a supervising authority looks like.

The person assigned to supervise us is not our enemy. But he or she is not our buddy either. Instead, that person's role is more like that of a manager who is there to help promote change while we are on supervised release. A power struggle with our supervising authority will only lead to self-defeat. It doesn't matter what that person's attitude is toward us. What matters is what we think of *ourselves*. It's our job to start taking more responsibility for our choices and our actions. Our supervising authority can help us stay on track, but it is up to us to take charge of our own lives.

Missed appointments, dirty urinalyses (UAs), and failure to appear in court or to report over the phone are all parole violations. If we don't want to violate parole, we need to follow directions, stay abstinent, keep appointments, and work hard. Then we'll succeed. Successfully completing supervised release depends on the choices *we* make, and only on *our* choices. Supervised release is only temporary *if* we follow the rules.

What Is the Role of a Supervising Authority?

A supervising authority will regularly meet with us to see how things are going and whether we are making progress toward our goals. He or she will ask questions about our recovery goals, listen to our concerns, and answer any questions we may have. More strict actions this person may take include testing us for alcohol and other drugs to make sure we remain abstinent, enforcing a curfew, investigating legal issues, making sure we follow the conditions of our release, and searching our home, vehicle, or person.

"Your PO is not your enemy. He is not out to send you back to prison. If you act like a criminal, sure— then he'll treat you like a criminal. But if you act cool, he'll work hard for you."

— LESTER

Duplicating this page is illegal. Do not copy this material without written permission from the publisher.

LIVING UNDER SUPERVISION • 27

If we do not follow the terms of our release, it will be our supervising authority's job to recommend or take appropriate action. Supervising authorities will record information to keep our case files updated and will stay in communication with other law officers. They can offer guidance and resources for additional support.

What Can We Expect from a Supervising Authority?

We can expect a supervising authority to maintain appropriate boundaries. If we do our best to follow the conditions of release, keep a positive attitude, and treat our supervising authority with respect, then we can expect fair treatment and respect in return.

Supervising authorities should explain rules, expectations, and directions clearly so that we are able to understand and follow them. They should talk to us about concerns they have and work with us to address those concerns. They should provide us with necessary forms and documents, along with guidance on how to complete them.

We can expect that our supervising authority will be accessible and supportive. This person is there to help us make changes in our lives with less supervision. He or she should listen to our questions and concerns and provide helpful feedback, including where to find additional resources.

What Can a Supervising Authority Expect from Us?

A supervising authority will expect us to maintain appropriate boundaries and will expect to be treated with respect. We should attend all scheduled meetings on time and should call ahead if we will be late. If we need to reschedule, we should provide an appropriate reason why that is necessary.

Our supervising authority will expect us to understand all of the conditions of our release *before* we are released and to ask questions when we don't understand. Any supervising authority will expect honesty from us, as well as a commitment to follow our recovery plan. This person will expect us to honor the condi-

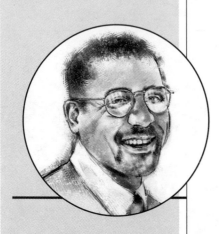

We can expect that our supervising authority will be accessible and supportive. He or she should listen to our questions and concerns and provide helpful feedback, including where to find additional resources.

tions of our release and follow all the rules—including ongoing testing for substance use and following a curfew. We are expected to cooperate with searches of our home, vehicle, or person at any time. We need to get permission for any changes related to our job or where we live.

It is especially important for those of us with co-occurring disorders to be honest with our supervising authority about our mental health. That includes being open and honest about medications, including how often and how much we take.

The following five tips will help us create a positive relationship with our supervising authority:

1. Be honest.
2. Discuss our problems.
3. Follow our relapse prevention plan.
4. Follow our supervising authority's directions.
5. Keep all appointments and commitments.

EXERCISE 2.4	QUICK REVIEW

Based on what you just read, fill in the blanks to complete the following statements.

1. It's _____ job to start taking more responsibility for our choices and our actions.

2. We can expect that a _____ _____ will be accessible and supportive.

3. Our supervising authority will expect us to understand all of the conditions of our release _____ we are released.

Tips for a Positive Relationship

1. Be honest.
2. Discuss our problems.
3. Follow our relapse prevention plan.
4. Follow our supervising authority's directions.
5. Keep all appointments and commitments.

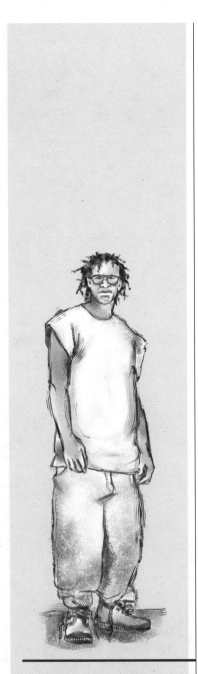

We all need help from time to time. But we need to ask for help, and we need to do it before problems get bigger.

How Can We Build a Positive Relationship with a Supervising Authority?

Adjusting to life after release will go much more smoothly if we take responsibility for building a positive relationship with our supervising authority. That starts with honesty and frequent communication. Supervising agents cannot read our minds, but they are there to help us. We all need help from time to time. But we need to ask for help, and we need to do it before problems get bigger. Choosing to be dishonest with our supervising authority puts us at risk for relapse. And we all know the risks associated with relapse.

Here are some other things we can do to help build a positive relationship with a supervising authority:

- Be open, honest, and willing to communicate— even if we've made a mistake.

- Stay abstinent from alcohol, other drugs, and criminal behavior.

- Ask questions to make sure we understand everything.

- Make a plan for change.

- Be flexible and patient with changes.

- Report as directed—be on time.

- Follow *all* conditions of release.

- Have a positive attitude—use positive self-talk.

- Set SMART goals.

- Attend support meetings.

- Keep a recovery-focused support system.

- Stay away from high-risk situations.

- Report any instances of trouble, such as arrest, within twenty-four hours.

1. List some of the things we can plan to do to build a good
   relationship with our supervising authority. Circle the
   ones you think are the most important.

   _____

   _____

   _____

   _____

   _____

2. Describe what might happen if we lie, run away, or ignore
   the conditions of our release.

   _____

   _____

3. List some positive ways to respond to requests from a supervising authority (such as obeying curfew or urinalysis).

   _____

   _____

   _____

   _____

   _____

Chad's Story

There's this mind-set coming in that I need to put on this persona that I'm not to be messed with—I'm strong, I'm not weak. A lot of these guys didn't have it anymore and they genuinely cared about not only the community they were in but the people that were in it. And that was a new experience for me. And the first thing that popped in my head was "I want some of that."

A lot of us were raised as men—we don't talk about things. We stuff that stuff down. We don't talk about our feelings, our emotions, what's bothering us. We don't cry. The more we talked about it, all of us together, the closer it brought us. So that we didn't stuff that stuff. We were basically learning that the ideas we were taught of what a man was weren't always correct. And so, we're learning basically how to be new men.

First and foremost, I'm gonna be asking my release planner what options are available for me where I have to parole. Setting up a relationship on a proper foundation of honesty, trust, mutual respect. A lot of the relationships that I had were built on what that person could do for me. Or what they could provide me. Knowing that I was very selfish in my relationships before has helped me now to see that relationships are a two-way street. I can't just be on the receiving end of what's being, you know, given. I have to also be the one who gives. I realized that in order for me to grow as a person, I have to have healthy people around me.

What to Do If We Relapse

Relapse is always a possibility—but it doesn't do any good to obsess about it. It is important to have a plan in place. Knowing what to do ahead of time and being prepared are the keys to recovery. We can go back on the recovery track again. We can talk immediately with someone supportive and abstinent, such as our supervising authority, sponsor or mentor, counselor, family member, friend, or spiritual leader. This person can help us return to working our recovery plan. We may also need professional help. And if things are really bad, we may need to enter a treatment program again.

If we do relapse, we need to take the following steps:

1. Stop and remove ourselves from the situation.
2. Ask for help.
3. Stay calm and forgive ourselves.
4. Renew our commitment to abstinence.
5. Analyze our relapse.
6. Make an immediate plan for recovery.

Remember that relapse is a process. Thoughts lead to cravings, cravings lead us to a decision, and sometimes that decision can lead us to relapse. It's important to pay attention to negative changes in our behaviors, attitudes, feelings, and thoughts. They could mean that the relapse process has already begun.

It's hard to ask for help. So instead of reaching out, we may try avoiding or running away from the situation. But that could make things worse. A supervising authority is there to help us, but we need to ask for help first.

When we ask for help, we accept that we're human. Human beings need each other to survive. Asking for help is a way to connect with another person. It sends a message of trust. And trust is the basis of a healthy relationship.

It takes strength to admit we screwed up and courage to get back on the road to recovery. We need to take positive action. The first steps are to stop using alcohol and other drugs, and to stop our criminal behavior. And we need to reach out for help.

EXERCISE 2.6	QUICK REVIEW

Based on what you just read, check *true* or *false* for the statements below.

1. Relapse is a process. Thoughts lead to cravings, cravings lead us to a decision, and sometimes that decision can lead us to relapse.

      True _____   False _____

2. Asking for help does not help build trust.

      True _____   False _____

Gary's Story

I told my PO that I was going to do an interview for this program. She said, "I'm not going to make you come down here and get a travel permit because you've been doing really good. So I'm just going to let you go, and let me know when you get back." And I said, "Okay."

So I took off, me and my daughter, and I was pulling a trailer. One of the lights on the trailer that I was pulling was out. So the police officer pulled me over, came up, and said, "I understand that you're on parole in Kansas." And I said, "Yeah." And she said, "Well I need to see your travel permit." And I said, "Well, you're out of luck, lady, because I don't got it."

And she said, "Where is it?" And I said, "I didn't get one because my PO said I was doing good, I didn't need to come down and waste my time getting it." So she said, "Well, the law is, you have to have a travel permit if you're out of the state of Kansas." And that is true, that is the law. So I said, "Well, I don't have it."

I did a thinking report and my immediate thought was, well, I'm going to jail anyways, so I might as well just go nuts. Then I thought, this isn't my fault. I just kept my composure and told her, "Okay, well, I'm going to need to get somebody to come and get my kid because I can't just leave her."

My uncle was working in Dodge City, Iowa, so he was there within about twenty minutes. I went to jail. I finally got ahold of my PO that afternoon and they said, "Okay, well, we're going to let you go. But you need to get a travel permit the next time you leave the state." And I said, "Okay, thank you." And I got out.

When I learned how to do the thinking reports, it helped a lot. That made me stop and realize that the things that I do and say are going to be different after thinking them thoughts. Being aware of my feelings about the situation, being aware of what I'm going to do . . . I'm in charge of that. I can control whether I yell at somebody; I can control whether I talk to somebody nicely; I can control any of that. And I didn't know that before.

continued

After I learned the thinking reports, I realized that I can help it. I do have an option to either get out of the situation or handle it the way it's supposed to be handled instead of just freaking out on people and getting mad and doing whatever. I was like, man, I can do this. I can behave or I can act like an idiot. So whichever one I decide to do is my choice, but it's been working to be good. So that's what I did.

I think the more you practice doing thinking reports in situations that are sticky, it's going to become easier and easier. Then pretty soon you don't even know you're doing it. You just do it because that's the way you do things.

Bottom line is, you were there, and you did what you did to get put in the situation that you're in now. It feels good to just say, "Yeah, it was me. I did it. And I will take my punishment." Own up to your mistakes, learn from them, and move on. There's no other way to do it.

EXERCISE 2.7   **REFLECTION**

1. Put yourself in Gary's shoes. What would you have done after being pulled over? Why?

   _____

   _____

   _____

2. Describe a time when you've successfully asked for and accepted help.

   _____

   _____

   _____

Duplicating this page is illegal. Do not copy this material without written permission from the publisher.

LIVING UNDER SUPERVISION • **35**

1. List a goal you have that is related to living under supervision after release.

   _____

   _____

2. How do you plan to achieve your goal?

   _____

   _____

3. What challenges might you run into?

   _____

   _____

4. How do you plan to overcome those challenges?

   _____

   _____

Chapter Summary

In this chapter we learned about living under supervision and explored how we feel about it. We learned about the role of a supervising authority after release and what we can expect from that person, as well as what he or she can expect from us. We explored how to build a positive relationship with a supervising authority and how important it is to ask for help. We also reviewed what to do in case we relapse. Finally, we identified a goal for living successfully under supervision.

Recovery Environment

By the end of this chapter, you will be able to	• describe how to manage risky environments • plan for a supportive recovery environment • identify housing goals related to housing after release • describe how to manage housing setbacks

A healthy recovery environment is one in which we can maintain a balanced lifestyle that is safe, abstinent, and as risk free as possible. A balanced lifestyle involves making sure we are fulfilled in all parts of our lives, including physically, socially, and environmentally. Everyone is different, so each one of us will balance our wellness differently. We can all get out of balance at various points in our lives, so maintaining a balanced lifestyle will look different for each of us.

Our supportive recovery environment should be cleared of obvious triggers, such as items related to substance use and crime (bottles of liquor, stolen property, etc.). We need to make sure it is as low risk as possible. It also needs to include an abstinent social support network. We've already learned we need support in recovery. We walk the recovery path together.

The Wellness Wheel: Eight Parts of Wellness

1. **Emotional** is about healthy relationships and keeping our feelings under control.

2. **Spiritual** is about having a sense of purpose and meaning in our lives.

3. **Intellectual** is about learning new things and using our creativity.

4. **Physical** is about exercising, eating healthy foods, getting enough sleep, and getting medical care when needed.

5. **Environmental** is about being around people or in places that are good for our health, well-being, and recovery.

6. **Financial** is about being okay with our money situation.

7. **Occupational** is about getting the most from our jobs.

8. **Social** is about connecting with supportive people.

WELLNESS WHEEL[1]

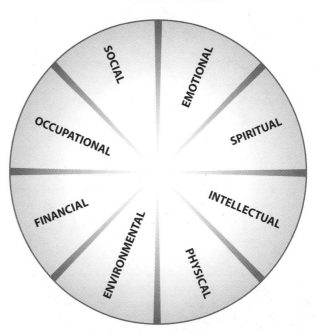

EXERCISE 3.1   **REFLECTION**

1. Describe three concerns you have about your recovery environment after release.

   a. _____

   b. _____

   c. _____

2. Describe what you think a good recovery environment would look like for you after release. Why do you feel that way?

   _____

   _____

3. What changes do you need to make in order to have a healthy recovery environment after release?

   _____

   _____

Safe, Sober, and Secure Housing

Where we live after release is very important. *Our housing must support our abstinence from substance use and criminal behavior.* But finding satisfactory housing can be difficult and complicated. As much as possible, we need housing that is safe, sober, and secure.

Long-Term Housing

We improve our chances at successful recovery when we find long-term housing that is safe, sober, and secure. We've learned about the risks associated with triggers, cravings, and high-risk situations. We need to feel safe and secure in our home environment. And it is very important that our home is free from substance use and criminal activity.

But housing can be expensive. And it takes time to go and look at places to live. It even takes time to get all the paperwork processed when you find the right place. Finding a new place to live is stressful, and our criminal history makes things even harder. Even if we find an affordable space that we like, we may get turned down. This can be really frustrating.

It helps to be flexible and patient when we are looking to find a place to live. And it helps to start thinking about housing in advance. There are things we can do now that will help us better understand what to look for when we are released. In fact, the first thing we may need to do is find a temporary place to stay while we look for something better. This is called *short-term housing*. The following questions address other housing considerations:

- How close do we need to be to work or school, our family, our recovery support group, our supervising authority, and so on?

- What can we afford? Are there additional costs?

- How much space do we need?

We improve our chances at successful recovery when we find long-term housing that is safe, sober, and secure.

- How will we get around (using public transportation, a car, etc.)?

- What is included in housing costs (laundry, kitchen, etc.)?

- How will we get to physical or mental health services?

- If we find a place that needs cleaning and repair work, do we have what we need to do that?

Short-Term Housing

When we get released, the first place we end up living may not be the greatest. It might be difficult for some of us to think our lives will get better if where we go after release isn't the place we'd hoped for. Again, it helps if we are flexible and patient, but our housing also needs to be approved by a supervising authority.

It is better to have *somewhere* to go rather than *nowhere* to go. And it is even better to think of more than one option, because then you can choose whichever is more safe, secure, and sober. Short-term housing is a place to stay while you look for better long-term housing. It is a step toward something better.

There are types of short-term housing that offer structured programs for people who have recently completed a treatment program. A sober living home, also known as a "halfway house," is somewhere ex-offenders and those in recovery can live in a community setting while they find work. Mutual support for abstinence can help us adjust to long-term recovery.

Sober living homes usually have strict rules for all who live there, including curfews and random drug testing. Independent recovery housing, also known as a "three-fourths house," is where the rules are less strict and residents have less community responsibility.

Not all sober living houses are safe, secure, and sober. We might come across criminal activity and alcohol and other drugs. In instances like this, we must consider whether there are any other housing options. If there are none, then we must consider ways to reduce the risks and support our recovery while we try to find better arrangements.

"When I realized I had a place to go every night, someplace I knew I could sleep and just be by myself, that was a big accomplishment. That's when I really believed I could make it."

— VERNON

Based on what you just read, fill in the blanks to complete these statements.

1. Our housing must support our _____ from substance use and criminal behavior.

2. We improve our chances at successful recovery when we find long-term housing that is _____, _____, and _____.

3. A _____ _____ home, also known as a "halfway house," is somewhere ex-offenders and those in recovery can live in a community setting while they find work.

EXERCISE 3.3   REFLECTION

1. List a few possible short-term housing options for you after release.

   _____

   _____

2. List some of the challenges that you might encounter with those short-term housing options.

   _____

   _____

3. List some ways you can overcome those challenges.

   _____

   _____

   _____

   _____

continued

4. List some of the things you would like in a long-term recovery environment.

_____

_____

5. List some ways you can start preparing now for a long-term supportive recovery environment after release.

_____

_____

Other Recovery Environment Considerations

What's Unhealthy?

When looking for a healthy recovery environment, it can be helpful to start with what is *unhealthy*. For example, we know that living with others who continue to use alcohol and other drugs is unhealthy for our recovery. We learned that a good relapse prevention plan uses both *avoidance* and *awareness* to manage our external triggers. And we learned that external triggers can include people, places, things, and situations. Problems related to physical, emotional, and mental health can also be strong triggers.

EXERCISE 3.4	REFLECTION

1. Who are some *people* you will need to avoid after release?

_____

_____

2. What are some *places* you will need to avoid after release?

_____

_____

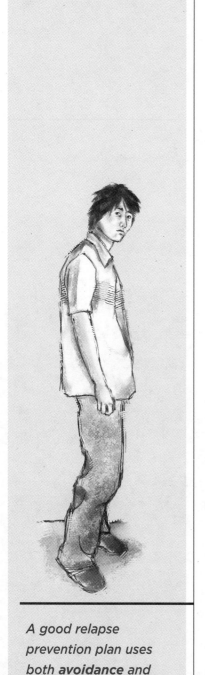

*A good relapse prevention plan uses both **avoidance** and **awareness** to manage our external triggers.*

3. Which *things* will you need to avoid after release?

_____

_____

4. Which *situations* will you need to avoid after release?

_____

_____

5. What are some ways you can be aware of your triggers so you can deal with them when they are unavoidable?

_____

_____

6. What are some physical, emotional, and mental health concerns you will need to address after release? How will you manage those?

   a. Physical: _____

   b. Emotional: _____

   c. Mental health: _____

Are Our Cultural Environments Healthy?

We can't be expected to live in a bubble after we get released. We might want to go to a movie with a friend, for example. We may want to work out at our community center. Some of us participate in spiritual communities. And there will be community, family, or other gatherings we'll want to attend on special occasions.

We all have unique cultural groups that we are involved with, such as our family, our faith community, and our neighborhood. We may be exposed to alcohol and other drugs in one or more of these environments. For example, we may see co-workers using alcohol and other drugs at work. People in our neighborhood may be involved with criminal activity. Community events might involve substance use, criminal behavior, or both.

Duplicating this page is illegal. Do not copy this material without written permission from the publisher.

RECOVERY ENVIRONMENT • **43**

We need to make sure our cultural environments support the positive changes we're making. In some cases, we may need to leave old communities and find new ones that better support our recovery goals. It is very important that we continue to practice good recovery skills and keep making healthy choices.

EXERCISE **3.5**   REFLECTION

1. List some cultural groups that you are involved with. Where do you meet?

_____

_____

2. List cultural events that will be challenging for you after release (family gatherings, religious festivals, a bowling league, etc.).

_____

_____

3. List some ways you can better manage those situations.

_____

_____

Is Our Thinking Healthy?

We have learned that our thoughts lead to feelings and that our feelings may lead to a behavior or action. Our old, distorted "stinking thinking" led us down a path to substance use and criminal behavior. But we've learned how to interrupt those faulty thinking patterns. We know how to make better choices now.

Part of planning for a healthy recovery environment after release is keeping our thinking healthy. We can think about our thinking as we make choices about our recovery environment. We need to avoid slipping into old thinking patterns and make sure we make the right decisions. Thinking Reports can help us take a deeper look at our thinking and make sure we are thinking in healthy ways.

| EXERCISE 3.6 | REFLECTION |

1. What are some ways your thinking might be challenged after release?

_____

_____

2. What are some things you can do to help yourself start thinking in healthier ways?

_____

_____

3. In what ways can a Thinking Report help your thinking?

_____

_____

How Do We Manage Setbacks?

We are likely to come across challenges and setbacks as we search for a healthy recovery environment. We will need to arrange an advance deposit to secure a place to live. Some of us have never rented before. We may run into restrictions due to our criminal record. No matter what challenges we face, we all experience them from time to time. We can start thinking now about how to prepare for them.

We need to make sure our cultural environments support the positive changes we're making. In some cases, we may need to leave old communities and find new ones that better support our recovery goals.

1. Imagine that you found a place where you would like to live, you took an afternoon off work to get a tour, and you filled out a rental application, only to be turned down. List some healthy ways to respond to this situation.

   _____

   _____

2. What are some other possible setbacks you might experience after release?

   _____

   _____

3. What are some healthy ways to overcome those challenges?

   _____

   _____

4. List some things you can do now to help prepare for future setbacks after release.

   _____

   _____

EXERCISE **3.8**   QUICK REVIEW

Based on what you just read, check *true* or *false* for the following statements.

1. A good relapse prevention plan uses both *avoidance* and *awareness* to manage our external triggers.

   True _____   False _____

2. It isn't necessary that our cultural communities support our recovery.

   True _____   False _____

3. Part of planning for a healthy recovery environment after release is keeping our thinking healthy.

   True _____   False _____

4. It does not help to prepare for setbacks.

   True _____   False _____

EXERCISE 3.9   **REFLECTION**

1. List one goal that you can start working toward now that relates to housing after release.

   _____

   _____

2. How do you plan to achieve this goal?

   _____

   _____

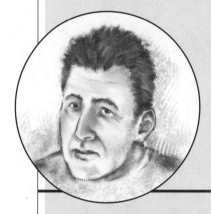

3. How will your cultural environments (neighborhood, work-space, place of worship, etc.) support this goal?

   _____

   _____

4. What challenges might you run into?

   _____

   _____

We have learned that our thoughts lead to feelings and that our feelings may lead to a behavior or action. We know how to make better choices now.

5. How do you plan to overcome those challenges?

   _____

   _____

   _____

   _____

Chapter Summary

In this chapter, we learned the importance of finding safe, secure, and sober housing after we're released. We explored the difference between short-term housing and long-term housing and discussed ways to manage some of the challenges and setbacks we might face when we look for a place to live. In addition, we recognized the importance of a healthy recovery environment, and we set a goal related to housing after release.

Support Network

By the end of this chapter, you will be able to	• describe what healthy support looks like • explain the differences between healthy and unhealthy relationships • describe the role cultural factors play in social support • plan for a healthy social support network after release

Recovery isn't an "I" language; it's a "we" language: we need to support our recovery with healthy, trustworthy relationships. That's why it's important to have a good support network in place all the time. Thinking about this now will help us to be better prepared for release.

Remember that healthy relationships have certain things in common, including these traits:

- Both people feel valued and respected.

- Both people trust one another.

- Both people feel safe problem-solving together.

- There are clear boundaries.

- There is clear communication.

- Both people feel emotionally connected to one another.

- Both people consider one another's point of view.

Duplicating this page is illegal. Do not copy this material without written permission from the publisher.

49

- Both people show understanding, acceptance, and forgiveness of one another.

- Both people recognize one another's accomplishments.

EXERCISE 4.1	REFLECTION

1. List some of the healthy relationships that you have.

_____

_____

2. What makes those relationships healthy?

_____

_____

3. What are some ways those healthy relationships will be helpful to you after release?

_____

_____

4. What are some concerns you have related to your support network after release?

_____

_____

It's important to recognize some of the key parts of our support network because our support network will change after release. Our long-term recovery will benefit from a variety of ongoing support. We're going to need different kinds of guidance and support from different parts of our support network.

Our support network includes these key people:

- **Therapist:** A therapist or counselor is a licensed professional who provides one-on-one counseling and support. Some therapists also lead group sessions when they think that will be helpful.

Our long-term recovery will benefit from a variety of ongoing support.

- **Sponsor or mentor:** A sponsor or mentor is someone who is abstinent and active in a recovery program. This is a person we can turn to in a crisis or call at any time.

- **Recovery support group:** A recovery support group is made up of individuals who are all in recovery and who support one another. They meet regularly and share contact information.

- **Spiritual advisor:** A spiritual advisor is someone we can share our story with and ask for help and spiritual guidance. Examples include a minister, priest, rabbi, imam, shaman, and guru.

- **Supervising authority:** A supervising authority is anyone who is assigned to supervise us after release. Examples include a parole officer, probation officer, and supervising agent.

- **Family:** A family is a system, or unit, that is made up of a number of individuals. Some of these people are related by blood; others are not.

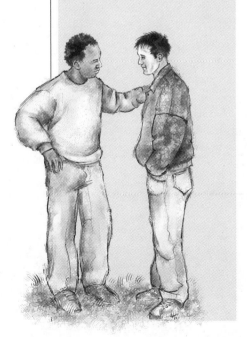

EXERCISE 4.2   **QUICK REVIEW**

Based on what you just read, fill in the blanks to complete these statements.

1. Healthy relationships have certain things in common, such as both people _____ one another.

2. Our long-term _____ will benefit from a variety of ongoing support.

3. A _____ or _____ is someone who is abstinent and active in a recovery program. This is a person we can turn to in a crisis or call at any time.

Duplicating this page is illegal. Do not copy this material without written permission from the publisher.

SUPPORT NETWORK • **51**

Healthy Family Support

Some family members can be great sources of support in our recovery. Others can be negative influences who encourage us to commit crimes and use alcohol and other drugs. We will need to figure out which family members are unhealthy for our recovery and which ones will provide healthy support.

Unhealthy family relationships have unclear boundaries that are not respected, and secrecy and shame keep people from talking openly about problems. We may not feel valued by these family members and may fear doing anything that goes against the "family code." Unhealthy family relationships might include going along with criminal behavior or using alcohol and other drugs. If our family members are not abstinent from alcohol, other drugs, and criminal behavior, then it may not be a good choice to be involved with them after release.

Healthy family relationships have good communication and a foundation of respect. We know what to expect from family members and have clearly established rules that are positive and consistent. We trust one another and feel valued. No family is 100 percent healthy or unhealthy; most families are somewhere in between. Different cultures have different family norms that may affect how we talk about things.

If our traditional family is not abstinent or not supportive of our recovery, we may need to find other people we consider to be family who support our recovery. Remember, family doesn't always mean blood relatives. Our understanding of family may change over time—bringing in new people and letting go of others.

Those of us with children also need to remember that our kids need parents. They need time, direction, and attention from us. They need and deserve to be respected as human beings, not as things or possessions. Our children are not our primary support in recovery. There are very few things in life that are more important than having a positive effect on the lives of our children.

Healthy family relationships have good communication and a foundation of respect. We know what to expect from family members and have clearly established rules that are positive and consistent. We trust one another and feel valued.

1. List people you consider to be family who will provide *healthy* recovery support after release.

   _____

   _____

2. List people you consider to be family who may be *unhealthy* to recovery and might be better to avoid after release.

   _____

   _____

3. How might your relationship with family members change after release?

   _____

   _____

4. What steps can you take now that will help you build healthy family relationships after release?

   _____

   _____

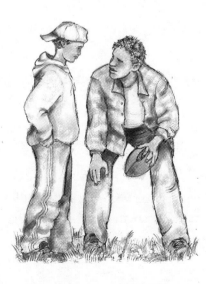

There are very few things in life that are more important than having a positive effect on the lives of our children.

Luis's Story

My first year it was kinda hard. I'd go to family functions and everybody's drinking, smoking, livin' the lifestyle. And a few of 'em were passin' stuff to me. I'm like, "Nope, no, no, I'm not—I'm tryin' something different. I'm tryin' something different."

They're still heavily involved in gang life, criminal activities, and all of the above. I love my family and I missed 'em so much when I was incarcerated. I tried to go see 'em and hang out with them a little bit. And you know, I had to start detaching myself and explaining to 'em, "I love you, but I love myself more. And you gotta go your way and I go my way."

I was hanging out with one of my uncles not too long ago. He used to be my role model. In a negative way. And now he's on a positive note, I'm on a positive note, so we hang out every weekend. And we laugh and joke about certain things we've been through. We'll be at a store and he'll be like, "Oh man, you can steal stuff from here real easy." And I just look at him and laugh like, "Ain't you too old for that? You don't wanna go get locked up again or nothing." And we'll laugh about it.

I used to break into cars, and there's times I walk by a car and I'll glance inside. And then I'll start laughing to myself. I know better now. I laugh about it, reflect on it, and thank God I'm on a different path.

EXERCISE 4.4 **QUICK REVIEW**

Based on what you just read, check *true* or *false* for these statements.

1. Some family members can be great sources of support in our recovery.

    True _____   False _____

2. It does not matter whether our family members are not abstinent from alcohol and other drugs or from criminal behavior—we can hang out with them anyway.

    True _____   False _____

3. Family only includes blood relatives.

     True _____   False _____

Healthy Social Support

Human beings are social. We need each other to survive, and we need each other to thrive. A healthy social support network is very important in our ongoing recovery. After release, it will be important to connect with others who support our abstinence and long-term recovery goals.

Trustworthy Relationships

Trustworthy relationships are healthy relationships. Our recovery efforts include thinking about our lives in a new way. Maybe others are pressing us to be more honest with ourselves. Maybe we're beginning to see ourselves in a new light. What matters is that we have honesty in our relationships, because that is what builds trust.

The hardest part of building healthy relationships that support recovery is letting go of our old lifestyle. That includes letting go of people in our lives who give us an excuse to keep using substances or committing crimes. We can change. We've already made important changes that are helping us make healthier choices.

We've learned about negative core beliefs, thinking distortions, criminal and addictive thinking patterns, and criminal and addictive tactics. All of these things can affect our social lives. To have healthy relationships, we need to be aware of them. Thinking Reports can help us stay on track. We've learned that we can change our thinking to help ourselves build healthier core beliefs. And healthier core beliefs will lead to healthier relationships.

Trustworthy relationships are healthy relationships.

1. What are some things you feel are important for building healthy relationships after release?

   _____

   _____

2. Other than your family, who are some people you have trustworthy relationships with?

   _____

   _____

3. What are some ways you can let go of or distance yourself from unhealthy relationships after release?

   _____

   _____

4. Discuss your answers to these questions with your group. List any additional helpful thoughts that came up during your discussion.

   _____

   _____

   _____

   _____

Support Groups

Being abstinent and supporting our own recovery is something we have in common with others who are abstinent and in recovery. We can grow our recovery support network by connecting with more people who are in recovery. Our similar experiences allow us to understand one another and support each other.

This program has given us a chance to participate in a recovery community. After release, we can expand our recovery support network by attending support meetings. Twelve Step groups offer lifestyle guidance and support for long-term abstinence and recovery. There are other recovery support groups and approaches, such as Secular Organizations for Sobriety or Walking the Red Road.

The best place to start is to attend a meeting. Most groups have websites that allow people to find meetings nearby or that list email or phone contacts. It can also be helpful to check local bulletin boards and telephone directories or to check resources at public gathering spaces. Many groups meet in community centers, churches, or schools.

Arriving early or sticking around after meetings allows people to talk more. Often people will go somewhere afterward to get coffee or decide to meet somewhere for a meal. These are opportunities to ask other people for phone numbers, email addresses, or another chance to meet later. It all starts with a willingness to meet new people.

To build a healthy relationship with someone else, get to know more about that person's interests. Reach out to that person, make plans with that person, and stay involved. If conflicts arise, make an effort to solve them together. Communicate often and openly.

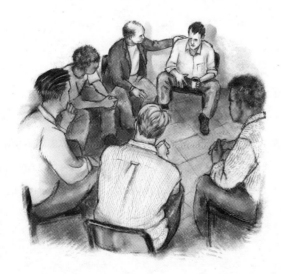

Based on what you just read, fill in the blanks to complete the following statements.

1. What matters is that we have _____ in our relationships, because that is what builds trust.

2. The hardest part of building healthy relationships that support recovery is letting go of our old _____.

3. We've learned that we can change our thinking to help ourselves build healthy _____ _____.

4. Twelve Step groups offer lifestyle guidance and _____ for long-term abstinence and recovery.

Other Recovery Support

Going to meetings isn't the only way to build our recovery network and help us commit to change. Having a good sponsor or mentor can help us as well. So can having a good therapist. Many people in recovery find support through a spiritual advisor. And we've already learned how our supervising authority can be a source of support. There are many other people who can be a part of our recovery network, but we need to give people the benefit of the doubt and reach out for support.

For those of us with co-occurring disorders or other mental health concerns, a therapist or psychiatrist may be a key part of our recovery. There are also special support groups for those with co-occurring disorders, those who take psychiatric medications, those in the LGBTQ community, and others. We are not alone in our recovery—we can find support groups that match our needs. But we may need help finding them, and it may take a bit of research. We must not be afraid to ask for help.

1. What are some ways that social support can help with your recovery after release?

_____

_____

_____

2. What are some ways you can ask others for help with recovery after release?

_____

_____

_____

3. What are some ways to find nearby recovery support groups after release?

_____

_____

_____

4. Discuss your answers with your group. List any additional helpful thoughts that came up during your discussion.

_____

_____

_____

_____

There are many other people who can be a part of our recovery network, but we need to give people the benefit of the doubt and reach out for support.

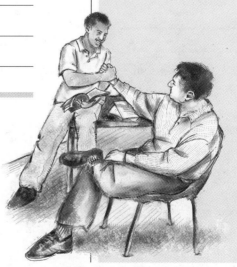

Duplicating this page is illegal. Do not copy this material without written permission from the publisher.

SUPPORT NETWORK • **59**

Healthy Sexual Relationships

Sexuality is part of everyone's lives and is part of our identity. Our past experience with sex affects our sexual relationships in recovery. And because many of us associate sex with alcohol and other drugs, sex can be one of our relapse triggers.

Reconnecting with previous sexual partners who use alcohol and other drugs puts us at high risk for relapse. Having sex with a prostitute is illegal, so that too involves high-risk behavior that may lead us to relapse. Both of these are examples of unhealthy sexual relationships. Unhealthy sexual relationships not only increase our risk of relapse, but they also increase our risk of unplanned pregnancy and sexually transmitted infections (STIs), also known as sexually transmitted diseases (STDs).

Healthy sexual relationships involve respect for our bodies and our emotions. They involve a close relationship with someone we care about—a relationship in which we don't just satisfy our own sexual needs and desires, but also respect a partner enough to help satisfy his or her needs too. Having a healthy sexual relationship is about making choices that keep us and our partner safe and healthy, both physically and emotionally.

A healthy sexual relationship is one in which *both* partners respect and maintain appropriate boundaries. It involves creating an emotional and physical connection to someone else—not pressure, threats, violence, or other aspects of relationship abuse. Honest communication is important. This means talking about sex *before* we have it.

When we are ready to date, which may take some time, we should look for a person who has the same positive qualities we look for in others within our support network. Dating does not need to involve alcohol and other drugs. There are many places to go and things to do that don't involve substance use. It is important that whomever we date takes our abstinence and recovery seriously.

Having a healthy sexual relationship is about making choices that keep us and our partner safe and healthy, both physically and emotionally.

1. What are some concerns you have about healthy sexual relationships after release?

   _____

   _____

2. What are some things you can do to help address these concerns?

   _____

   _____

3. What are some ways you can build healthy sexual relationships after release?

   _____

   _____

4. What are some things you can do on a date that don't involve alcohol, other drugs, or criminal activities?

   _____

   _____

Healthy Cultural Support

We are a part of a lot of different social groups. We may participate in neighborhood events, we may play sports with a group of people, or we may be involved in a religious community that worships and celebrates holidays together. Each group has its own culture. The word *culture* describes a group's way of life that includes beliefs, values, traditions, and customs.

Since we are in recovery, we can say we are involved in recovery culture. If we keep up with modern art, music, television, and news, then we can say we are aware of popular culture. In fact, we may participate in many different cultures, such as family culture, national culture, ethnic culture, and work culture.

It is helpful for us to think about our cultural groups before we are released. We need to make sure that the cultural groups we participate in are supportive of our abstinence and recovery. That may mean we will have to avoid or deal with triggers and high-risk situations. It may mean changing the way we participate so that it is healthier for our recovery. Our cultural groups can be an important part of our support network, as long as they help us to remain abstinent.

EXERCISE 4.9	REFLECTION

1. What are some of the cultural groups that you identify with?

_____

_____

2. What are some healthy ways you can participate in these cultural groups after release?

_____

_____

3. What are some of the challenges you might face with these cultural groups after release?

_____

_____

4. In what ways can you overcome the challenges you listed?

_____

_____

_____

_____

1. List a goal related to building a healthy support network
   after release.

   _____

   _____

2. How do you plan to achieve your goal?

   _____

   _____

3. What challenges might you run into?

   _____

   _____

4. How do you plan to overcome those challenges?

   _____

   _____

Chapter Summary

In this chapter we learned what healthy relationships look
like and covered some of the different types of recovery support we'll need after release. We thought about some of the
key parts of our support network. We learned about healthy
family support, healthy social support, healthy sexual relationships, and healthy cultural support. We considered how
we might prepare ourselves for healthy relationships in each
of these areas after release. Finally, we set a goal around
building a healthy support network after release.

Duplicating this page is illegal. Do not copy this material without written permission from the publisher.

SUPPORT NETWORK • **63**

Occupational Goals

By the end of this chapter, you will be able to	• define what *personal occupational success* means
	• explain the difference between short-term and long-term employment
	• discuss employment assistance options
	• plan for healthy occupational goals after release

In chapter 3 of this workbook, we talked about a balanced lifestyle in all of the different areas of our lives that are represented in the Wellness Wheel. One of the areas has to do with occupational wellness. The word *occupation* refers to the activities and business that someone is involved in.

An occupation could refer to a job, but it could also mean school or community service work. For example, a plumber is someone who works with water pipes, valves, and tanks. A student is someone who studies, attends classes, and does research. A volunteer is someone who helps others without expecting payment.

After release, we will need to find a way to earn money. What we decide to do will be different for all of us. Some of us will plan to get a job right away. But others of us may decide to go to school or to volunteer because the jobs we want require us to finish school or complete volunteer training before we can be hired.

Duplicating this page is illegal. Do not copy this material without written permission from the publisher.

65

1. Describe what occupational success means to you.

   _____

   _____

2. Describe how you feel about making changes to gain occupational wellness.

   _____

   _____

3. List some resources that might help you better plan for occupational wellness after release.

   _____

   _____

When we think about a job, one of the first things that comes to mind is how much we'll be paid. While money is important, it is not the only thing to consider. Job satisfaction is also important. If we plan to work full time, we can expect to spend at least forty hours a week on the job. That's a lot of time to spend somewhere, so it is a good idea to try to find a job we enjoy.

Short-Term Employment

It might help to understand the difference between short-term employment and long-term career planning. Earlier we talked about the difference between short-term housing and long-term housing. That same idea also applies to our occupation. When we first get released, we might have to take a job that's not in the career field or industry of our choice, or we may accept a job that is not at our desired level just so we can start making some money.

Just like with housing, it helps to be flexible and patient. Short-term employment is better than not having a job. It allows us to earn money in the short term. And that's a step in the right direction while we look for something better.

Our criminal history may make finding a job even harder than it already is. It is challenging to find employers who will hire someone with a criminal background. We may have trouble accepting a minimum-wage job, a part-time job, or a job doing something different from what we want to do. We may think it would be easier to get money illegally instead of earning money in an honest-paying job. That thinking will only get us into trouble.

It was our criminal behavior that put us in our current situation. Our crimes hurt both us and others. As we prepare for release, we must remind ourselves that the money we made illegally came at a hefty price. Our commitment to abstinence and recovery shows that we plan to do things differently after release. Honest-paying, short-term employment is much better for our recovery than anything illegal. And right now, our recovery is priority number one.

Getting a dream job will not happen on our first try. We can think of short-term employment as a stepping stone on the path to long-term occupational success. Like all good things in life, success requires a bit of work. It may take time for us to figure out where we want to be. And once we do, it's going to take work to get there.

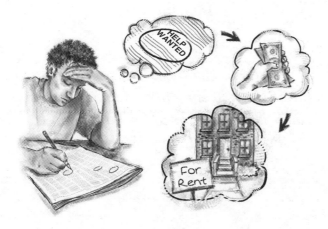

"There are no short-cuts to any place worth going."

— BEVERLY SILLS

1. What are some of your concerns related to finding a job after release?

_____

_____

_____

_____

2. What are some businesses where you might be willing to look for work soon after release?

_____

_____

_____

_____

3. What are some things you can do now that will help you find work after release?

_____

_____

_____

_____

Like all good things in life, success requires a bit of work. It may take time for us to figure out where we want to be. And once we do, it's going to take work to get there.

Ezra's Story

My entire youth I sold weed. I never really had to do anything. I could always figure out some kind of angle to get at some money. There was a guy that at one point in time owed me some money from a long, long time ago. I called him to get some weed and ended up robbing him.

My whole lifestyle was trying to hustle up money. Obviously to get high. Every day probably cost me a minimum of five hundred dollars just to be awake. That criminal lifestyle was revolving around drugs. In order to get five hundred dollars a day, you can't go work at a job. It's very hard to make five hundred dollars a day every day.

I was on work release at the end of my sentence and started working for this guy for eight dollars an hour, twenty hours a week. I would get on the bus at like 6, 7 in the morning and I would really work to 11 p.m. every day. But I only got paid for twenty hours a week at eight dollars an hour. I knew I had to put my hours in. I had to work a lot. I had that motivation of not going back to prison. I don't want to have anything to do with that. And if I could sit in a cell all day long, I might as well go try to make money all day long. I set goals for myself and I make sure I follow 'em. I read 'em every day.

Anybody who complains that it's not worth the hard work—any sort of stress out here is way better than the stress in there. So if I can have my tough times out here, it's cool. I made a decision to not go back. I've been out about two and a half years. I own five or six rental properties now. We have rooms for rent for guys outta prison systems, out of group homes, treatment centers. That's kinda my way of giving back.

Every year you live fast out there you might do two in slow. Think how slow prison is. You might have a couple years up, but you're gonna have a couple years down. Better to have a couple years even.

Applying for Jobs

Applying for jobs is a job in itself. It takes time, hard work, and patience. It also requires determination and toughness. We are not going to be offered every job we apply for, but it's still tough to get rejected. We need to be patient—with determination, we *will* find a job. There are things we must do first, however.

Getting a job involves searching for job openings, building a resume, filling out job applications, writing cover letters, and going to job interviews. Learning about these important steps will help us with our long-term occupational goals.

Searching for Jobs

It is easy to feel overwhelmed at the beginning of a job search. Some of us might even be applying for a job for the first time. Where do we even start? Step one is to start looking.

You can find a lot of jobs online. Most companies have job listings on their websites. In fact, there are websites with the single purpose of listing job opportunities. You can use filters to narrow down your search. Try searching online using different key words. See what results you get and follow links that look promising.

You can also find jobs in local newspapers, both online and in print versions. Of course, shops and other businesses also put Help Wanted signs in their windows, so it's sometimes helpful to just walk or drive around to see what's available. It can also help to ask people if they know of any opportunities. They might have recommendations for us, and they might be able to recommend us to others. Keep an open mind and explore all options.

Building a Resume

Some businesses may ask us to turn in a *resume* in order for us to be considered for the job. A resume is a brief overview of our work experience, education, training, skills, volunteer experience, and contact information. Try and include sections for each one of those areas on your resume. Create headings for each one and use that as a starting point.

Being incarcerated makes it difficult to list recent work history. But many of us have worked, volunteered, and studied during our incarceration. Putting together a resume is an opportunity for us to call out the things we *do* have to offer.

While we want to be honest in what we say about ourselves, it does help to think about how we say things in a resume. For example, instead of just listing "inmate" or leaving a gap in our employment history, consider listing skills you learned while incarcerated, such as cleaning tasks, kitchen duties, and other work you performed. Also, think about what skills you have that others might not have, such as speaking more than one language. Writing a resume gives us a chance to be positive and creative with how we present ourselves.

It is helpful to include experience that relates to the jobs we apply for. For example, if we want to apply for a job as a cook, it will be helpful to list any experience we have preparing food and cleaning up a kitchen. The point of a resume is to show why we would be a good fit for the job and what we can bring to the job. Include words from the job description in your resume—that will show similarities between what the employer is looking for and what we have to offer. When employers screen applicants, they often look for key words from the job description in the applicant's resume or cover letter—if we don't include the right key words, we might not make the first cut.

We can use job descriptions to our advantage. For example, a job description often lists skills the company is looking for— good information to address in our resume and cover letter. We can also pick out key words from the job description to include in our resume or cover letter. For this reason, it might be helpful to update our resume each time we apply for a job so that it is specific for that particular job and business. There are good examples of sample resumes online, and we can use those to help us build our own.

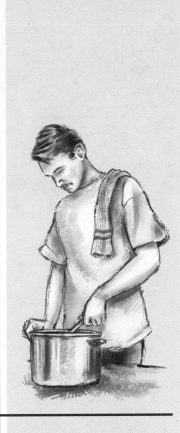

It is helpful to include experience that relates to the jobs we apply for. For example, if we want to apply for a job as a cook, it will be helpful to list any experience we have preparing food and cleaning up a kitchen.

Based on what you just read, fill in the blanks to complete the following statements.

1. Getting a job means searching for job openings, building a _____, filling out job applications, writing cover letters, and going to job interviews.

2. Most companies have job listings on their _____.

3. It might help to _____ your resume each time you apply for a job.

EXERCISE 5.4   REFLECTION

1. What are some ways you can look for jobs after release?

   _____

   _____

2. What are some experiences you've had as an inmate that could help you find work after release?

   _____

   _____

3. What are some things you might include on your resume?

   _____

   _____

   _____

   _____

Filling Out Job Applications

Instead of asking for a resume, some businesses will ask us to fill out a job application. And some businesses will ask us to fill out a job application *and* provide a resume. Employers often need to keep records for those who apply, and job applications are often part of that record keeping.

A job application will require a lot of the same information that can be found in your resume, such as your name, employment history, education, and contact information. It may ask for other things as well, such as references. In some businesses, job applications may still ask about criminal history. It helps to know our rights in the states where we live. It may be frustrating to include this information at such an early stage in the application process, but we will be expected to answer questions like this honestly.

A job application and a resume are often used for different purposes, so it is often helpful to provide both. Ask the employer about the job application process to make sure you submit all the required paperwork.

In today's world, many job applications are completed online. In fact, applications might even be scanned and filtered by computers before they are passed on to hiring managers. That is why it is very important to understand and complete the entire application process. It would be a shame to miss out on a job opportunity simply because we didn't fill out the application correctly or because we missed a step in the process.

In today's world, many job applications are completed online. That is why it is very important to understand and complete the entire application process.

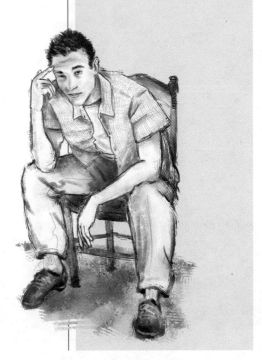

Writing Cover Letters

A cover letter is a personal message we send to a potential employer. It gives us the chance to say more about why we want the job and why we might be a good person to hire. A cover letter is an opportunity to introduce our resume and our job application. And it is one more opportunity to tell a potential employer about ourselves.

It can be hard to neatly and briefly sum up our skills and work experience, but it is worth the effort. First impressions are important, and a cover letter serves as a first impression. It gives us room to say a little bit more about ourselves than we can fit in our resume, and it allows us to do it in a personal and memorable way.

Again, it can be helpful to use words from the job description in our cover letter to show that we have the qualities the employer is searching for. We can also include achievements that set us apart from others. Just as sample resumes are online, good examples of cover letters may be found online that we can use to help us write our own.

EXERCISE 5.5	REFLECTION

1. Who are some people who might make good references for you on a job application?

   _____

   _____

2. What are some things you might include in a cover letter that aren't on your resume?

   _____

   _____

   _____

Interviewing for Jobs

If an employer is interested in your resume or job application, his or her next step is to contact you. Often first contact with you will be a brief phone call in which someone from Human Resources will ask basic questions to confirm the information you provided in your application and resume. The next step will be an interview. An interview usually involves meeting face-to-face, although some employers may choose to do an interview by phone instead. Some companies may even do video interviews. No matter how the interview takes place, it is an opportunity for the employer to get to know more about you, and it is a chance for you to find out more about the job.

We may be asked some difficult questions in an interview, including information about our criminal record. To show that we are trustworthy, it is important to be honest and up front. However, we don't need to go into great detail. We can also use the interview as an opportunity to talk about what we've learned and some of the positive changes we've made.

It may be helpful to do a practice interview beforehand. We can ask someone we know if he or she will pretend to be an employer, or we can interview ourselves in the mirror. If we think about how we might answer questions or what we might say, we can feel more confident in an actual interview. Here are some other tips to help us prepare for interviews:

- Read about the company beforehand (what it does, where it is located, what it sells, etc.).

- Think about how you will introduce yourself and how you might answer questions. The first question is often, "Tell me about yourself."

- Think about questions you can ask to show that you are interested and have done some preparation.

- Clean up and dress nicely to make a good first impression.

- Show up early to make sure you are not late.

- Stay calm (try and relax, make eye contact, don't fidget, etc.).

- Don't share too much—stick to information about yourself that relates to the job.

- Shake hands with everyone you meet.

- Send a thank-you letter within twenty-four hours after your interview.

Employers often receive so many applications for a job that they don't have time to respond to every person who applies. Some companies send out an email confirming that your application has been received, but it is common to not hear anything else. This happens to everyone. Do not take it personally, and don't get discouraged. Keep a positive attitude and stay motivated and determined. Above all else, don't apply for one job and then sit back and wait for a response. Keep applying and interviewing until someone offers you a job.

EXERCISE 5.6	QUICK REVIEW

Based on what you just read, check *true* or *false* for these statements.

1. A job application and a resume are one and the same, so it is never required to provide both.

    True _____   False _____

2. A cover letter serves as a first impression.

    True _____   False _____

3. Getting called for an interview means you already got the job.

    True _____   False _____

Working under Supervision

We have discussed some of the challenges related to living under supervision, and we learned some ways to overcome those challenges. We are likely to face some of those same concerns when we start a new job.

Having a job usually means having a boss. Because of this, we can expect to have someone regularly review our work and give us feedback on how well we are doing. It is a good idea for us to start thinking now about how we might handle working under supervision after we are released.

Jobs can be stressful, so it will be helpful for us to plan ways we can deal with stress on the job. It is also natural to occasionally run into conflict with others at work, so we can also think about ways we might reduce tension if conflict happens on the job. Negative core beliefs can affect our work performance, so it is important for us to pay attention to our thinking. Positive thinking may help us stay out of trouble and keep us from getting fired.

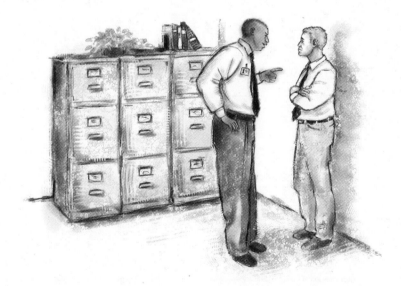

It is natural to occasionally run into conflict with others at work, so we should think about ways we might reduce tension if conflict happens on the job.

Complete a Thinking Report using a past conflict with a work supervisor as the event.

Thinking Report

1. Event _____

_____

2. Thoughts _____

_____

3. Feelings _____

_____

4. Behavior _____

_____

5. Core Beliefs _____

_____

6. Alternative Thoughts _____

_____

7. Alternative Behaviors _____

_____

Thinking Distortions _____

_____

Thinking Patterns _____

_____

Tactics _____

_____

Long-Term Employment

In the long run, we hope to find a job that we find fulfilling. No job comes without problems, but it helps if we can find a job that we enjoy going to for forty hours a week. And we can start doing some career planning now.

A *career* is a field of occupational pursuit. That can refer to any occupation. For example, it can mean a skilled tradesperson, such as a carpenter, a baker, or an electrician. It can also mean a learned professional, such as a teacher, a scientist, or a medical professional. We may be ready to start a career path right away, depending upon which field we choose.

However, some careers will require certification training, some will require a diploma and/or a degree, and some will require experience through volunteer work. Because of this, long-term career planning might require us to take classes or volunteer our time before we can even apply for a job.

Where short-term employment focuses on our immediate needs, long-term employment focuses on our ongoing job satisfaction. A career isn't just about money; it's about finding a job we enjoy. And that takes a bit more planning.

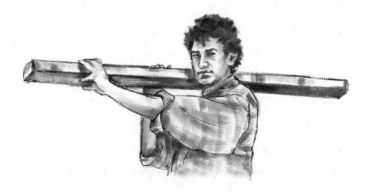

A positive, hard-working attitude can give us the drive we need to achieve occupational success.

Working Hard

We've learned what an important role our thinking plays in our lives. Negative core beliefs and thought patterns not only affect our job performance; they can also destroy our career goals. But a positive, hard-working attitude can give us the drive we need to achieve occupational success.

When we stay focused on achieving our goals, we can face challenges head-on and overcome them. A healthy and productive life is within reach as long as we continue to work hard. Success is not something reserved for lucky people only, but it takes work and dedication to stay on course even when times get tough. Here are some other things that will help us get ahead in our jobs and careers:

- honesty
- trustworthiness
- responsibility
- cleanliness
- good communication
- flexibility
- motivation
- loyalty

One way to keep our drive to succeed is to feed that drive. It's good to want to move up in a job or a company. It's good to look for opportunities for advancement. Think about things that will help you get promoted: are there things you can do now that will help you achieve those things? Thinking about the future can help us stay motivated, and that is exactly the type of drive we need to get ahead.

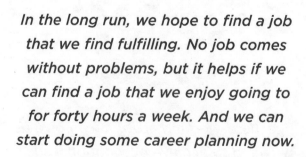

In the long run, we hope to find a job that we find fulfilling. No job comes without problems, but it helps if we can find a job that we enjoy going to for forty hours a week. And we can start doing some career planning now.

EXERCISE 5.8   REFLECTION

1. What are some of the challenges that have kept you from an honest career path in the past?

    _____

    _____

    _____

2. What are some new career challenges you might face after you are released?

    _____

    _____

    _____

3. What are some things you can do now to help prepare for those challenges after release?

    _____

    _____

    _____

4. What are some things you can do after release to avoid or overcome those challenges?

    _____

    _____

    _____

When we stay focused on achieving our goals, we can face challenges head-on and overcome them.

Tyrone's Story

I started setting out plans for how I was going to gain some employment when I got out. I wanted to have some type of skill or trade when I came home from prison. I stayed focused and got certified within six months and that's normally a year program.

We were planning on moving from Minnesota to Seattle, but my wife figured that was too far away from her family. And so we looked for places that had a lot of welding jobs. And Duluth fell on the table for us as a viable option.

When you step out of prison and you find yourself alone and you find yourself needing help, you're quick to run back to what is familiar. But if you don't have ready access to what is familiar, then you start looking for new ways.

I've got six felony convictions. And so, with my record, a lot of people and companies will not give me the opportunity to even get my foot in the door, to even get an interview. Instead of me quitting or taking on the attitude to blame other people, I decided to be persistent.

I showed up at a bunch of companies. I mean, I showed up earlier than the employers would show up, and I'd be there and say hi with a friendly smile and ask, "Hey, have you got time for an interview?" A person really has to be determined.

I believe wholeheartedly there's hope for gentlemen who are in prison and in jail and suffer from addiction. There is a great hope for them. The other day I was sitting down with my wife and kids at the dinner table and we was going over what we're thankful for. And my seven-year-old daughter told me that she's thankful that I love her no matter what. I never thought I would hear something like that. It keeps me going.

Setting SMART Goals

A successful career takes some advance planning. One of the easiest things we can do to help plan our careers is to set goals. It may be helpful to start with some smaller goals and then move on to bigger goals.

Remember, it's a good idea to set goals that are SMART:

- **S**pecific
- **M**easurable
- **A**chievable
- **R**elevant
- **T**ime-bound

One example of a small SMART goal that we can set for ourselves to start our career planning is to research three career paths that interest us within the next week. After we have collected information on three possible career paths, we can set some small SMART goals related to each one. Each career is different, so the goals we set for ourselves in order to succeed will be different. What's more, career paths may change quickly and unexpectedly.

For example, if a company we are working for gets sold to another company, the owners may decide to relocate their offices. In that case, we may need to either move to a new city or look for a different job. If there aren't any other companies that do the same type of work where we live, then we may want to make a career switch. Our skills may be a good fit for another career, but this is one example of why it helps to be flexible with career goals.

A successful career takes some advance planning. One of the easiest things we can do to help plan our careers is to set goals.

SMART Goals

- **S**pecific
- **M**easurable
- **A**chievable
- **R**elevant
- **T**ime-bound

1. What are some long-term career paths that you may be interested in learning more about?

_____

_____

2. What are some SMART goals related to the career paths you identified?

_____

_____

3. What are some of the things you will need or will need to do to achieve the SMART goals you identified?

_____

_____

4. What are some things you can do now that will help you to achieve your long-term career goals after release?

_____

_____

5. Ask others in your group for feedback related to your career goals. List some of their suggestions.

_____

_____

Training, Education, and Volunteering

We are all lifelong learners. Learning is really about being open to life and being curious about the world we live in. In fact, if you stop to think about it, you've probably learned something new very recently.

There are many different ways of learning. We can learn from watching an informational video, reading a book, or taking an online course. Some other ways we can learn include on-the-job training, volunteering, or an internship. Or we might attend a vocational school or college. Again, it helps to research some career paths that interest us. By doing so, we will learn about the education or training required in those fields.

Some occupations will require schooling, while others will not. Some will require experience that we can get by volunteering instead. We usually don't have to pay money to volunteer, but we do need to invest our time. Training and schooling will cost both time and money, although we may qualify for scholarships and student loans.

We are all lifelong learners. Learning is really about being open to life and being curious about the world we live in.

Randy's Story

I came to prison with a second-degree murder charge. I was fortunate that they had a college program. And I took advantage of that college program and I got my associate arts degree. I wrote to the foreman and told him I'd like to get back into the electrical shop. I knew I had to find something of a trade that was marketable when I got out. A couple of guys that worked there were master electricians, and they gave me books and stuff so I could learn it. So I learned an awful lot while I was there and took advantage of it.

Since I got out of prison, I got a job at a company that does cell towers. I worked as an apprentice again because I didn't have my license. I worked there for a while digging trenches, putting pipe into the ground. Now I passed my journeyman's test and got my license. Next year, I'll take my test for my master's.

It's been rewarding. I learned to be patient—to work for it and to make a plan, make a goal. I'd never planned before I went to treatment or looked at goals or anything like that. It was just whatever happens, happens. Now I lay out goals, I study. There's a lot of jobs out there that you can get if you set a goal and a plan that you can conquer.

Duplicating this page is illegal. Do not copy this material without written permission from the publisher.

OCCUPATIONAL GOALS • 85

Based on what you just read, fill in the blanks to complete the following statements.

1. One of the easiest things we can do to help plan our careers is to set _____.

2. _____ paths may change quickly and unexpectedly.

3. We are all lifelong _____.

4. Some occupations will require _____, while others will not.

Occupational Assistance

Even with what we've learned so far about employment after release, looking for a job can still seem overwhelming. Fortunately, there are a number of resources available to help us. And we may want to seek additional guidance from our support network, both before and after release. Some of these resources might even be available through counselors before we are released. Here are some additional helpful resources:

- **Career counseling assessment:** This tool measures our interests, skills, personality traits, values, goals, and more. It can help us figure out jobs and careers that might be a good fit for us. It can also help us to set short-term and long-term occupational goals. Some of the assessments can be found online, but we can also get help with them at career service centers.

- **Vocational rehabilitation and workforce centers:** These centers offer a variety of services and resources to help with finding employment. They can help connect job seekers with local employers, offer assistance with resumes, help with job searches, teach people where and how to search for jobs, offer training, assist those with disabilities, and provide access to telephones, copy machines, and computers.

- **Federal and state bonding programs:** These government services open doors for those whose backgrounds make it difficult to find a job. They offer no-cost fidelity bonds (insurance) to employers who hire people with criminal histories. They also help individuals who are leaving treatment or correctional facilities to find jobs.

- **Work Opportunity Tax Credit (WOTC):** This is a federal tax credit that is offered to employers as an incentive to hire people who have been incarcerated and others struggling to find jobs. More information is available through the United States Department of Labor's Employment and Training Administration.

EXERCISE 5.11   REFLECTION

1. List an occupational goal you have for yourself after release.

_____

_____

2. How do you plan to achieve your goal?

_____

_____

3. What challenges might you run into?

_____

_____

_____

_____

continued

4. How do you plan to overcome those challenges?

_____

_____

Chapter Summary

In this chapter, we were introduced to the occupational part of overall wellness. We learned the difference between short-term and long-term employment. We also learned some of the basics of applying for jobs: how to search for jobs, build a resume, fill out job applications, write cover letters, interview for jobs, and work under supervision. And we learned some tips for long-term career planning, including working hard and setting SMART goals. We received information on training, education, and volunteer work. Finally, we learned about occupational assistance and set an occupational goal for after release.

6

Free Time

By the end of this chapter, you will be able to	• describe how thinking can affect recreational activities • explain healthy ways to manage social events • describe ways to deal with boredom and loneliness • plan healthy ways to spend free time after release

Our decisions about how we spend our free time are critical to our recovery. Having time to do things we want to do is likely something we are looking forward to after release. But having free time also creates some problems for us. Some of the choices we've made in the past have gotten us into trouble. For this reason, it may be good for us to do a bit more planning around how we will spend our time.

The idea of planning our free time may not make sense to us. But remember that certain people, places, things, and situations can be triggers for us. And we've learned that triggers can lead to cravings, and cravings can lead to relapse. Because of this, we can see that planning how we spend our time is actually helpful to our recovery. And what's helpful for our recovery will also help us prepare for the reentry process.

1. What are some ways you can spend free time after release that support your recovery?

_____

_____

2. What are some concerns you have related to free time after release?

_____

_____

3. List a few people you enjoy spending time with who are abstinent and support your recovery.

_____

_____

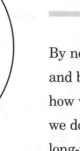

Our thinking patterns affect the ways we behave around others.

By now, we are familiar with how core beliefs, thoughts, feelings, and behaviors are all related to one another. We understand that how we think affects how we feel, and that in turn affects what we do. Our thinking, therefore, will play an important role in our long-term recovery and in helping us to stay abstinent.

Negative core beliefs can cause distorted thinking, while healthy core beliefs can strengthen our relapse prevention efforts. It's not easy to replace negative core beliefs with healthy ones, and it doesn't happen overnight. It is something that requires ongoing work, and this will be especially important after release.

Our thinking patterns affect the ways we behave around others. As a reminder, here are the distorted thought patterns, described earlier, that could show up in our social interactions:

- **extreme thinking** (all-or-nothing thinking), when we view everything as one extreme or another

- **overgeneralization** ("always" or "never" thinking), when we think that if something happened once or twice, it must always be true

- **personalization** (making everything about us), when we only see things from our point of view and think everything that happens around us is all about us

- **magnification and minimization** (making something seem greater or smaller than it really is), when we take an event out of context and blow it out of proportion, or we downplay its impact or significance

- **jumping to conclusions** (assuming something without getting all the facts), when we think we know something and make snap decisions with no evidence

- **selective focus** (looking at only one small piece of what happened), when we focus only on certain parts of a story or situation

- **concrete thinking** (stubborn, "I know what's right" thinking), when we focus on details but don't understand the message behind them

- **actor versus observer** (thinking we are never at fault or responsible for our behavior), when we believe situations just happen to us and we don't take responsibility for our actions

- **closed thinking** (no one can tell us differently), when we don't listen or trust new information

- **emotional reasoning** (making conclusions based on our feelings), when we believe that our feelings are facts

It is easy to slip into old ways of thinking. For example, we might think about our upcoming release as though it were the end of our treatment and incarceration. But we know better. We still have supervised release, and we know that there is no end to our recovery.

In some ways, our recovery is just beginning. We will have more free time after release, and we will have more freedom. But that is why it is especially important to pay attention to our thinking. Relapse prevention and recovery support will be most critical in the days just after our release.

Triggers and High-Risk Situations

During our free time, we'll run into triggers and cravings, which can push us into our old behaviors of committing crimes and using alcohol and other drugs. Not all of us have the same triggers or cravings, but we all have some. One person might react to a memory. Another person might be triggered by a certain smell. Walking into a place that serves alcohol might trigger someone else.

It is normal to experience triggers, but they are different for everyone. It's really important for us to understand our own triggers, especially as we prepare for release. When we know what triggers a craving, we can take steps to avoid or deal with that trigger. And when we deal with our triggers in healthy ways, our cravings will get weaker. Over time, the cravings can even disappear.

Trigger ➔ Thought ➔ Craving ➔ Decision ➔ Relapse

After release, we are bound to run into triggers and high-risk situations. But thinking about them in advance gives us an advantage—we can figure out coping strategies we can use to manage the triggers and high-risk situations. Two common coping strategies are awareness and avoidance. *Awareness* means noticing triggers. *Avoidance* means staying away from known triggers.

It can be easy for us to gain awareness of some triggers and high-risk situations. For example, being around alcohol and other drugs is not a good idea. If we are aware of that, we can avoid places where these drugs will be present, such as a bar or a party. But not all triggers or high-risk situations are that obvious. Finishing a day of work, parenting children, and even just walking down the street can also be high-risk situations.

- A **trigger** is an event that sets off a desire to do something unlawful or to use alcohol and other drugs.

- **Internal triggers** involve the thoughts, emotions, or sensations (physical or mental) we have that spark a craving.

- **External triggers** include the people, places, things, and situations we encounter that spark a craving.

- A **craving** is the urge we feel after we experience a trigger. Cravings are tricky "mind messages" that try to convince us that we need a drink, that we need a drug, or that we need to do something unlawful.

- A **high-risk situation** is any situation in which we are strongly tempted to use substances or commit a crime.

Based on what you just read, fill in the blanks to complete these statements.

1. Negative core beliefs can cause distorted thinking, while healthy core beliefs can strengthen our _____ _____ efforts.

2. Relapse prevention and _____ _____ will be most critical in the days just after our release.

3. Trigger ➔ Thought ➔ Craving ➔ _____ ➔ Relapse

4. Two common coping strategies are _____ and avoidance.

People

It is also a good idea to think about the people who pose a risk to our recovery, because we will likely want to try and avoid them. Examples include someone who may commit a crime or use alcohol or other drugs around us, a friend or relative who might pressure us to return to old patterns of behavior, or people we used to commit crimes with.

Instead, we need to think about abstinent people in our lives who will help support our recovery after release. We may want to reach out to them before we are released and make plans to get together. It will also be helpful to think about ways we can make new abstinent friends. We might want to research recovery support groups in the area we plan to live after release and make plans to attend meetings.

> *It is a good idea to think about the people who pose a risk to our recovery, because we will likely want to try and avoid them.*

Places

We need to be aware of places we should avoid after release. We may need to change our routes and routines. For example, it will not be a good idea for us to go to a bar, a place where we used to use or buy drugs, a party where we know there will be alcohol and other drugs, an area of town where we used to commit crimes, or a place where we used to meet up with fellow gang members.

Instead, we need to consider places that will be healthy recovery environments for us. Of course, we will want to have fun after release. But we'll want to think about places where we can have sober and crime-free fun. We will want to find new hangouts that are safe and pose a low risk.

Things

There are certain items that we will want to stay away from after release. Obvious things include alcohol, other drugs, and weapons. But there are other things we will want to avoid that are less obvious triggers, such as prescription bottles, something we wore when we committed crimes, and music we listened to while using. We may even want someone in our support network to help us make sure our future housing is free from high-risk items.

It is possible to find new things to replace the old ones. We may want to replace the weapon we used to carry around with a sobriety medallion. We may want to add a list of emergency support contacts to our wallet. Or we may want to get a basketball or a guitar to encourage ourselves to play.

Situations

We will also encounter risky situations after release, and some will be difficult to avoid, for example, family holiday celebrations, neighborhood barbecues, having sex, or even just watching TV.

We will want to think about how we can manage high-risk situations in ways that support our recovery. For example, we may decide to skip high-risk events or ask someone else who is abstinent to attend them with us.

EXERCISE 6.3	REFLECTION

1. List some external triggers you will want to avoid after release.

   a. People:

   _____

   _____

   _____

   b. Places:

   _____

   _____

   _____

   c. Things:

   _____

   _____

   _____

   d. Situations:

   _____

   _____

   _____

continued

2. List some external influences that will be healthier for your recovery.

a. People:

_____

_____

b. Places:

_____

_____

c. Things:

_____

_____

d. Situations:

_____

_____

_____

Thoughts and Feelings

After release, we are going to need to pay very close attention to our negative thoughts, negative feelings, and negative core beliefs. Some examples include feelings such as anger, fear, guilt, and shame or thoughts like "It's a dog-eat-dog world," "I deserve special treatment," "It won't matter if I just have one drink," or "Insurance will pay for whatever I steal."

We also might need to be wary of some *positive* feelings, such as excitement, happiness, pride, amusement, and lust. Thoughts like "I can stay sober at a party," "I can commit small crimes and keep it under control," and "I can cook with alcohol without drinking it" are risky.

Instead, it will be helpful for us to focus on *positive affirmations,* or thoughts we can repeat to ourselves that can help us to change the way we see ourselves and the world around us. Some examples include "I can change," "Easy does it," or "Progress, not perfection." Replacing negative thoughts with positive affirmations may seem silly or stupid, but doing so actually helps replace our negative core beliefs with healthy, positive ones.

Physical Problems

We may run into physical problems after release. For example, we may break a bone, need dental work, or experience sleeplessness. If this happens, we will need to find a doctor or dentist who understands addiction and be honest with that person about our past substance use.

We can find alternative ways to manage physical problems that will support our recovery. For example, we can find non-addictive pain relievers that do not cause intoxication, or we can try massage treatment or acupuncture. Some alternative approaches will help with both physical and emotional problems, such as meditation, relaxation exercises, or talking through problems with someone from our support network.

Emotional and Mental Health Problems

We may run into situations, such as the loss of a loved one or a custody battle for children, that lead to emotional problems. Some of us might also need to manage mental health problems after release. If we have co-occurring disorders, it will be important for us to find a therapist and keep regular appointments. We may need to make sure we regularly take medication. We might also need to find special support groups that understand and accept our mental health concerns.

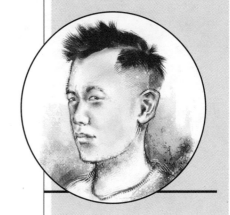

*it will be helpful for us to focus on **positive affirmations,** or thoughts we can repeat to ourselves that can help us to change the way we see ourselves.*

1. List some internal triggers you may run into after release.

    a. Thoughts and feelings:

    _____

    _____

    b. Physical problems:

    _____

    _____

    c. Emotional and mental health problems:

    _____

    _____

2. List some healthier ways you can prepare for and manage internal triggers.

    a. Thoughts and feelings:

    _____

    _____

    b. Physical problems:

    _____

    _____

    c. Emotional and mental health problems:

    _____

    _____

Complete a Thinking Report using a past high-risk event
or a time when you experienced a trigger.

Thinking
Report

1. **Event** _____

   _____

2. **Thoughts** _____

   _____

3. **Feelings** _____

   _____

4. **Behavior** _____

   _____

5. **Core Beliefs** _____

   _____

6. **Alternative Thoughts** _____

   _____

7. **Alternative Behaviors** _____

   _____

Thinking Distortions _____

_____

Thinking Patterns _____

_____

Tactics _____

_____

Sober, Crime-Free Fun

Being abstinent doesn't mean we cannot have fun. But it does mean we need to be thoughtful about what activities we choose to do. Some of our old activities involve triggers that may be risky to our recovery.

EXERCISE 6.6	REFLECTION

1. List some things you would like to do for fun after release.

_____

_____

_____

_____

2. Look at the things you just listed and cross out any that involve triggers or high-risk situations.

There are sober and crime-free activities we can have fun doing instead, as long as those activities don't involve triggers for us. Some examples include going to a park or museum, taking a class, going out to eat, shopping, going to an auto show, and participating in a recovery walk.

As we get further along in our recovery, we will realize that we can have fun without committing crimes and without alcohol and other drugs. Enjoying sober activities can help us find new hobbies—things we regularly do that help maintain our recovery, such as biking, reading, fishing, and exercising.

It will be important for us to have fun independently as well as with others. And to have fun by ourselves, we'll need to make sure we feel good about ourselves and enjoy our own company. We must learn to forgive ourselves for our past mistakes and value ourselves instead for the changes we've made to better our lives.

We cannot have good relationships with other people until we know how to be a good friend to ourselves. For this to happen, we need good self-esteem—respecting ourselves and believing in our worth and abilities. A balanced approach to wellness can help build our self-esteem and is an important step toward improving our relationship with ourselves.

We can also consider people we admire: why do we look up to them? What can we can do for ourselves that will help us be more like those people? Our values tell us what we want to live by and live for. They are the silent forces behind many of our decisions and actions. Think about people we admire and what values they have, and then think about making positive changes to our own values that could help our recovery.

By regularly looking at the positive things in our lives, we practice having an "attitude of gratitude." That attitude can help us realize that we don't want to screw up those good things by using alcohol and other drugs or by doing something that will get us into trouble. Instead, we focus on what's going well. Thinking about what we are thankful for helps us to avoid triggers that put us at risk for relapse.

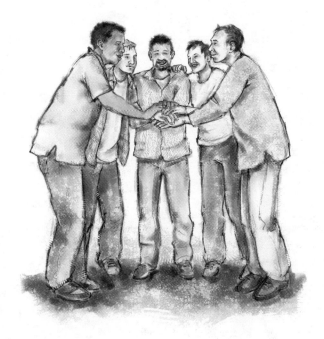

As we get further along in our recovery, we will realize that we can have fun without committing crimes and without alcohol and other drugs.

Based on what you just read, check *true* or *false* for the statements below.

1. Being abstinent means we cannot have fun.

   True _____   False _____

2. Enjoying sober activities can help us find new hobbies.

   True _____   False _____

3. We cannot have good relationships with other people until we know how to be a good friend to ourselves.

   True _____   False _____

4. Thinking about what we are thankful for does not help us avoid triggers or avoid relapse.

   True _____   False _____

Helping Others

In chapter 5, we discussed how volunteering is something we can do to help us find a job. But it is also something we can do to help ourselves. Helping other people can make us feel good. And it's something we can do that supports our abstinence and recovery.

Addiction and criminal behavior have caused us to spend a lot of time thinking about ourselves. Part of changing our thinking involves considering the well-being of others. We've learned about the importance of social support in recovery, but social support isn't just important to those in recovery. There are a lot of people who need help and a lot of organizations that need volunteers.

Many volunteer opportunities are community events that are free from criminal activity and substance use. Attending public outreach events like these and meeting other volunteers can help us remain abstinent. Not only do these events provide a healthy way to spend our free time, but they offer us a chance to expand our social support network.

Many people think of volunteer work as a way of giving back, but the volunteers also benefit from it. It is a sober, crime-free activity, it provides a healthy recovery environment, it gives us the chance to meet new people who can help support our recovery, and it feels rewarding.

EXERCISE 6.8	REFLECTION

1. What are some things you can do now to help plan for healthy free time after release?

    _____

    _____

2. What are some groups or events that you can get involved with after release that don't involve substance use or crime?

    _____

    _____

3. What are some ways you can encourage yourself to stay active and involved in the things you just listed?

    _____

    _____

Boredom and Loneliness

Boredom and loneliness are two very high-risk internal triggers that can lead to relapse. If we have nothing to do, we might be tempted to use substances or commit crimes. It's normal when we look back at our days of using alcohol and other drugs and committing crimes to focus only on the exciting parts. It's not fun to think about the parts that got us in trouble with loved ones and the law—the things that got us where we are today.

Boredom is a choice, but it can sneak up on us. We need to plan ahead to avoid boredom and loneliness. Planning healthy activities will help us avoid risky behavior and live a more positive life that is focused on recovery.

It can be helpful to pay attention to the times of day that we know are especially hard—the times when we most often think about substances and criminal activity. Then we can schedule something positive to do during those hours.

The Importance of a Daily Routine

Planning our day ahead of time can give us structure and purpose and will help prevent boredom and loneliness. Breaking our days down into manageable pieces helps keep us from feeling overwhelmed. A healthy routine also reduces temptation and stress, which in turn reduces our chances for relapse.

We've learned that a balanced lifestyle is important, so we need to schedule time for sleep, healthy meals, exercise, meditation, and sober fun in addition to our daily tasks. The Wellness Wheel in chapter 3 can help us achieve balance in all areas of our lives. Many people get in the habit of making a to-do list at bedtime with tasks and activities for the next day. Others benefit from making a twenty-four-hour schedule.

We need to avoid large gaps of empty time in our schedule, since that can cause us to become bored or lonely. To avoid criminal and addictive thinking, we need to fill our time with constructive, healthy, sober activities. At the same time, we shouldn't overcompensate and get too busy, as that can cause stress-related triggers.

Boredom is a choice. We need to plan ahead to avoid boredom and loneliness.

1. Try planning your own twenty-four-hour schedule for your first day after release. Make sure to include at least eight hours for sleep and to avoid gaps of empty time while you are awake.

12:00 a.m.	
1:00 a.m.	
2:00 a.m.	
3:00 a.m.	
4:00 a.m.	
5:00 a.m.	
6:00 a.m.	
7:00 a.m.	
8:00 a.m.	
9:00 a.m.	
10:00 a.m.	
11:00 a.m.	
12:00 p.m.	
1:00 p.m.	
2:00 p.m.	
3:00 p.m.	
4:00 p.m.	
5:00 p.m.	
6:00 p.m.	
7:00 p.m.	
8:00 p.m.	
9:00 p.m.	
10:00 p.m.	
11:00 p.m.	

2. Discuss your schedule with your group and list additional suggestions or concerns.

_____

_____

Cultural Events

We are likely to spend some of our free time after release attending events and participating in activities within our cultural communities. While cultural groups may be an important part of our lives and our support network, we need to make sure that these events will not turn out to be high-risk situations for us or involve triggers.

There are many different types of cultural events, and all of us belong to different cultural groups. However, some cultural events present common concerns for all of us, especially holidays and special occasions. These can be stressful and can involve powerful emotions. For this reason, they can be especially risky for us, since stress and emotions can be triggers that increase our risk of relapse.

Putting a plan in place before we head into these activities and events can help us to better manage any risks that might come up. Here are a few tips to help us plan ahead:

- Ask someone we trust (for example, an abstinent relative or friend) to go with us.

- Let our sponsor, mentor, or another support person know where we'll be so we can have an escape plan in place if anything threatens our recovery. We should keep emergency contact information handy for times of crisis.

- Practice role-playing using potential risky situations so that we can be better prepared for them if they actually happen.

- Excuse ourselves from risky situations or choose to attend support meetings instead of attending risky events in the first place.

- Be proactive by suggesting activities that support recovery in advance. This could be a simple suggestion like requesting no alcohol and other drugs at an event, or it could be a suggestion for something much different, such as volunteering together at a homeless shelter.

- Let people know we're in recovery so there is no pressure to participate in substance use or criminal activity.

Putting a plan in place before we head into activities and events can help us to better manage any risks that might come up.

Based on what you just read, fill in the blanks to complete the following statements.

1. Boredom and _____ are two very high-risk internal triggers that can lead to relapse.

2. Planning our day ahead of time can give us structure and _____ and will help prevent boredom and loneliness.

3. There are cultural events that present common concerns for all of us, such as _____ and special occasions.

4. Putting a _____ in place before we head into these activities and events can help us to better manage any risks that might come up.

1. List a goal for yourself that supports healthy ways to spend free time after release.

   _____

   _____

2. How do you plan to achieve your goal?

   _____

   _____

3. What challenges might you run into?

   _____

   _____

4. How do you plan to overcome those challenges?

   _____

   _____

Duplicating this page is illegal. Do not copy this material without written permission from the publisher.

FREE TIME • **107**

Chapter Summary

In this chapter, we reviewed how our core beliefs, thoughts, feelings, and behaviors are all related to one another, and we discussed how important they are to our long-term recovery. We reviewed the dangers associated with triggers and high-risk situations, and we discussed some specific ways to better prepare ourselves to manage these after release. We learned about the importance of sober, crime-free fun and of the risks that boredom and loneliness can present to us. We explored relapse prevention strategies, including the importance of planning a daily schedule, and we discussed healthy approaches to cultural events. Finally, we set a goal that supports healthy ways we can spend free time after release.

Health and Wellness

By the end of this chapter, you will be able to	<ul><li>define what balanced wellness looks like after release</li><li>plan healthy physical wellness after release</li><li>plan healthy emotional wellness after release</li><li>plan healthy spiritual wellness after release</li></ul>

A balanced approach to wellness means being healthy in the many different parts of our lives.

If we try to find ways to better balance the different parts of our lives, we increase our chances of remaining abstinent and strengthening our recovery. A balanced approach to wellness means being healthy in the many different parts of our lives.

Everyone is different, so each one of us will balance our wellness differently. Some of us already exercise. Some of us already meditate or pray. Some of us already have a good support system. But practicing better balance will improve our overall health and make reentry easier. Balancing healthy habits can lead to positive feelings about ourselves, others, and the world around us.

1. What are some of the ways you currently support *balanced* wellness in your life?

    _____

    _____

2. What are some of the things you currently do for *physical* wellness in your life?

    _____

    _____

3. What are some of the things you currently do for *emotional* wellness in your life?

    _____

    _____

4. What are some of the things you currently do for *spiritual* wellness in your life?

    _____

    _____

Physical Wellness

When we think of physical wellness, most of us think of exercise. And that is certainly an important part. But there is more to physical wellness than just having a fitness routine or being active. Our bodies send us signals that we can pay attention to. By listening to what our bodies are telling us, we can learn to take a more balanced approach to overall physical wellness.

Our bodies send us signals that we can pay attention to.

Let's use exercise as an example. It is good to be routinely physically active. But being inactive can also be good. The goal is to create a balance somewhere in between. While a good workout can feel good, we can actually damage our bodies if we push too hard too fast. Sometimes we need to apply ice to sore legs rather than go for another run.

We shouldn't ignore our bodies when they beg for attention, and this applies to all kinds of physical wellness. For example, we can often tell when we are hungry or sleepy. But there are times when we don't stop to eat or we stay up later than we should. That can lead to foul moods and poor performance at work. When we pay more attention to our physical needs, we can improve the way we feel. And that is the key to physical wellness.

Exercise

Each of us has our own idea of what an exercise routine looks like. Some of us might practice yoga or martial arts; others might like a sport such as tennis or basketball. Still others might like to run or lift weights. There are multiple ways to exercise, and that means we can likely find something that we enjoy doing.

If possible, it is good to exercise on a regular basis. We may have developed regular exercise habits while incarcerated, but the trick is to keep a regular routine *after* we're released. It will be harder after release because we will have more things that we will be responsible for, such as finding a place to live and work and building a recovery support network. But staying active can help us reduce stress and cope with challenges.

It is good to set goals and work toward them one day at a time. For example, being overweight not only presents a health risk for us; it also means we probably don't feel our best. It may help to set small goals that we can achieve rather than setting impossible ones. After we reach that small goal, we can set another one. With each goal we achieve, we'll feel a sense of accomplishment for the progress we're making.

There are multiple ways to exercise, and that means we can likely find something that we enjoy doing.

Even small efforts can make a big difference—like taking the stairs instead of an elevator, parking farther away from the entrance to a building, or walking or biking to work instead of driving or taking the bus.

We also don't need to join a gym or hire a personal trainer. We can find home workout routines in fitness magazines, learn yoga techniques by watching online videos, and find fitness sites that provide guidance for free.

EXERCISE 7.2	QUICK REVIEW

Based on what you just read, check *true* or *false* for the statements below.

1. When we talk about physical wellness, we're really talking about exercise.

    True _____   False _____

2. When we pay more attention to our physical needs, we can improve the way we feel.

    True _____   False _____

3. If possible, it is good to exercise on a regular basis.

    True _____   False _____

4. We should join a gym if we want to achieve physical wellness.

    True _____   False _____

Nutrition

Eating healthy is a key part of physical wellness, and many people with substance use disorders have poor diets. What we eat will affect our bodies, including our moods, thoughts, and feelings. Therefore, it will be important for us to eat well after we are released in order to stay healthy. That includes eating regular meals, not skipping meals, and making healthy choices about what we eat.

If we are overweight, changing our diet is one of the best ways to be healthier. We can benefit from eating small, healthy portions at regular mealtimes throughout the day. Learning about healthy portions and recommended guidelines will help us to eat a balanced diet. That will include fresh, healthy foods like fruits and vegetables. We may also need to cut down on junk food and caffeine.

We can also set small nutritional goals. Instead of making extreme commitments for long periods of time, we should start instead with small changes every day or every week. For example, cutting down on our sugar intake for a few days is more realistic than trying to cut all sugar out of our diet for the next six months. We can do some of our shopping at a farmer's market. We may be able to sign up for the federal Supplemental Nutrition Assistance Program (SNAP), which offers nutritional assistance to low-income individuals and families. There also may be local programs that can offer similar assistance.

If possible, we can try to eat at home so that we can better track what goes into our meals. It may also help for us to track what we are eating and how much we consume. A dietician or nutritionist can provide assistance, but we can also find advice online and in health magazines. There are even government recommendations that provide guidance. A nutritious diet can make a big impact on our physical wellness, especially when we combine it with a healthy exercise routine.

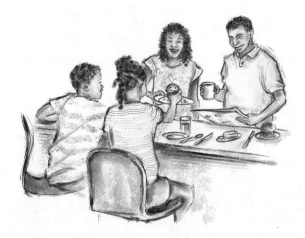

If possible, we can try to eat at home so that we can better track what goes into our meals.

1. What are some physical activities that you enjoy?

   _____

   _____

2. What are some ways you can work these activities into your regular routine after release?

   _____

   _____

3. What are some positive eating habits that you currently have?

   _____

   _____

4. In what ways do you plan to improve your nutrition after release?

   _____

   _____

Sleep

Ask people how much sleep they need in a night, and the answers are bound to vary. The National Institutes of Health recommend that adults get seven to eight hours of sleep each night to be well rested.[1] However, many people don't get the recommended amount of sleep. In fact, many people claim they can get by on much less, but that is a myth that research has proven to be false.

In today's fast-paced world, Americans work more hours per week than people in many other countries around the world. But it's not just work that is keeping people up at night. Entertainment is available around the clock, especially in today's digital age. Whether it's due to work or fun, people are generally getting less sleep than they should.

Sleep is good for our physical health and wellness, and we should try to get the recommended amount every night. According to the U.S. Department of Health and Human Services,[2] getting the recommended amount of sleep can help us

- avoid getting sick
- maintain a healthy weight
- reduce stress
- improve our mood
- think clearly
- get along better with others
- avoid injury
- lower our risk for serious health problems such as diabetes and heart disease

Winding down at the end of the day can be an important step in helping us to fall asleep faster and more easily. There are many different ways to relax before bed, so it is a good idea to find some that work for us. Some common methods include reading a book, taking a bath, and drinking a cup of hot herbal tea.

There are also things we can avoid, such as exercising too close to bedtime and using electronic devices in bed. Exercise will increase our heart rate, and the blue light from electronic screens can disrupt our internal clock that helps us get sleepy.

EXERCISE 7.4	QUICK REVIEW

Based on what you just read, fill in the blanks to complete these statements.

1. What we eat will affect our bodies, including our moods, _____, and feelings.

2. A nutritious diet can make a big impact on our physical wellness, especially when we combine it with a healthy _____ routine.

continued

3. The National Institutes of Health recommend that adults get _____ to _____ hours of sleep each night to be well rested.

4. Winding down at the end of the day can be an important step in helping us to _____ _____ faster and more easily.

"I think about it this way: I don't brush my teeth, I get a cavity. It gets bad. It hurts. Suddenly I need six hundred dollars. Hmm. Where can I get six hundred dollars?"

— JOE

Preventative Care

Many health problems may be prevented if we regularly keep tabs on our own physical wellness. The idea behind preventative care is that routine maintenance will keep us healthy and prevent bigger health problems down the road. For example, if we regularly brush our teeth, floss, and schedule dental appointments, then we will be much less likely to get a cavity.

We can compare preventative health care to a car—if we never change the oil, then we are bound to run into engine problems down the road. We can replace a car if it breaks down, but we can't replace our bodies. This is why preventative health care is so important. Regular exercise, good nutrition, and the right amount of sleep are all important examples of preventative care.

A yearly physical exam with our doctor is also part of preventative care, and so is a routine teeth cleaning every six months at the dentist. There are guidelines for how often we should schedule checkups with health care providers, but those guidelines depend on what we're having checked. Think about a car once more—we change the oil more frequently than we get new tires.

It's a good idea to get some things checked more frequently than others. For example, we should have our weight checked regularly to make sure we're not heavier than average, our blood pressure checked regularly to help ensure we don't have a stroke, and our cholesterol checked regularly to help ensure we don't have a heart attack.

The first step in preventative care is to make sure we have health insurance. Most full-time jobs offer health insurance through the company, but there are other ways to get insurance. This is an important consideration as we prepare for release, and we may need help learning more about it. We can discuss it with our therapist before release, and we can also ask those in our support network for help.

Another option is to visit a local public health center or to contact the Health Resources and Services Administration (HRSA). There are HRSA programs available all across the country, and they can help uninsured people, people in rural areas, and others who have difficulty accessing health care to receive medical services.

EXERCISE 7.5	REFLECTION

1. What are some healthy things you do to help yourself fall asleep at night?

_____

_____

2. What arc some things you plan to do after release to make sure you regularly get a full night's rest?

_____

_____

3. What are some of the things you currently do that you think of as routine health maintenance?

_____

_____

4. What are some of the things you plan to do after release to make sure you practice good preventative health care?

_____

_____

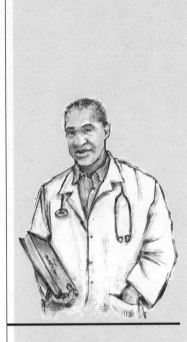

A yearly physical exam with our doctor is also part of preventative care, and so is a routine teeth cleaning every six months at the dentist.

Sexual Health

Earlier we discussed how healthy sexual relationships involve a physical and emotional connection with a potential sexual partner. It is also important to learn about personal sexual health—things we can do to help ourselves prepare for sex after release.

Personal cleanliness is an important part of self-care that prevents infection and illness. It is also an important part of our social life, which includes sexual health. Our personal appearance affects the way others see us and the way we feel about ourselves. That in turn affects our entire social life, but it is especially important when we are sexually active with someone. Some basic things we can do for personal cleanliness include

- brushing our teeth twice a day
- flossing our teeth once a day
- taking a bath or shower
- clipping our fingernails and toenails once a week
- washing our sheets and towels every week
- cleaning our bathroom, kitchen, and bedroom regularly
- washing our hands after going to the bathroom, before handling food, after changing a diaper, after playing with a pet, and before and after taking care of someone who is sick

Another important part of sexual health is getting tested for and protecting ourselves against sexually transmitted infections (STIs). People usually get an STI through sexual contact. Some STIs affect our health more seriously than others, but if we plan to be sexually active, we should take steps to protect ourselves.

The safest way to avoid getting an STI is to not have sex. But if we choose to have sex, there are ways we can be safe. We can get vaccinated against some STIs by visiting our doctor. Meeting with our doctor also gives us the chance to discuss any other sexual concerns we might have, such as anxiety about sex, problems getting an erection, body image issues, or concerns about pornography or sexual addiction.

The safest way to avoid getting an STI is to not have sex.

The more people we have sex with, the more we risk getting an STI, which is why having sex with a prostitute is risky. Using protection during sex, such as using a condom or a dental dam (a thin sheet of latex used for oral sex), will help us avoid getting an STI. Using protection is also an effective method of birth control, which protects against unwanted pregnancy.

The safest way to have sex is to be sexually active with only one person. It is important for both people to get tested *before* having sex to make sure neither one has an STI. Being sexually active with only one partner is a good way to make sure that both partners are safe and healthy, both physically and emotionally. And that is an important part of a healthy sexual relationship.

| EXERCISE 7.6 | QUICK REVIEW |

Based on what you just read, fill in the blanks to complete these statements.

1. The idea behind preventative care is that routine _____ will keep us healthy and prevent bigger health problems down the road.

2. The first step in preventative care is to make sure we have _____ _____.

3. Personal _____ is an important part of self-care that prevents infection and illness.

4. The safest way to avoid getting an STI is to not have _____.

Duplicating this page is illegal. Do not copy this material without written permission from the publisher.

HEALTH AND WELLNESS • 119

Emotional Wellness

Another important part of a balanced lifestyle is emotional wellness, which has to do with communicating our feelings, taking care of ourselves, managing stress, and for some, managing mental health. We already know that our feelings influence how we behave. Understanding our emotions better can help us to act in more positive ways.

Communicating Feelings

Sometimes it is hard to figure out exactly how we feel, and putting those feelings into words can be even harder. On top of that, sharing our feelings with others can make us feel vulnerable and uncomfortable. But the more we understand and talk about our feelings, the more comfortable it will feel.

Earlier in this workbook, we talked about the importance of having trustworthy relationships. If we trust someone, we will likely feel more comfortable talking about our feelings with that person. Talking through our feelings will help us to feel better, so it is important to find people we trust.

Some feelings are easier to identify than others. For example, we can often feel ourselves getting hungry or getting angry. But other feelings are not as obvious. For example, feeling angry might actually be our way of dealing with deeper feelings such as loneliness or fear.

It can help if we write down our feelings. Keeping a daily journal of our feelings might help us to think about them more clearly. It can also help us find the right words to express how we feel. Writing those words in a journal will also make it easier to share them with someone we trust.

When we learn to communicate our feelings, we take responsibility for them. And that can help us improve what we do in response to our feelings. If we take responsibility for our feelings, we take responsibility for our actions—an important part of reentry.

1. Explain how you feel right now.

_____

_____

2. Talk about your feelings the next time you meet with your group. Then explain how it felt to talk through your feelings.

_____

_____

3. Who are some people you trust that you can share your feelings with after release?

_____

_____

4. What are some things you can plan to do to better communicate your feelings after release?

_____

_____

Taking Care of Ourselves

The first step in taking care of ourselves is getting to know ourselves better. We can start by keeping track of our feelings in a journal, but we may also want to keep track of other things. For example, it can help to write down some of the things that help us feel calm and safe, or some of the things that help lift our spirits.

Staying positive and focused is an important part of emotional wellness, and it will be an important part of successful reentry after release. We all do things to help ourselves feel comfortable and calm, whether it's taking a walk every day, enjoying a quiet moment with a hot cup of coffee in the morning, or talking on the phone with a loved one.

We learned earlier about the importance of a recovery support network after release. It's helpful to point out that our support network also strengthens our emotional wellness. There are people we turn to in times of need, and it may be worth noting who those people are.

It's also important for us to spend time alone. We know ourselves better than anyone else, and that makes us our own best friend. Recognizing and building a positive relationship with ourselves will only help us with our long-term recovery.

EXERCISE 7.8 **QUICK REVIEW**

Based on what you just read, check *true* or *false* for the statements below.

1. Talking about our feelings will not help our emotional wellness.

    True _____   False _____

2. Taking responsibility for our feelings leads to taking responsibility for our actions.

    True _____   False _____

3. The first step in taking care of ourselves is getting to know ourselves better.

    True _____   False _____

4. Spending time alone is unhealthy for our emotional wellness.

    True _____   False _____

We know ourselves better than anyone else,
and that makes us our own best friend.

Managing Stress

Life after release will be stressful. Preparing for release is stressful. The truth is, we will always have stress in our lives. How we manage our stress is important to our emotional wellness and our overall wellness.

As we know, stress can be a trigger for us—and triggers increase our risk of relapse. We've discussed ways to deal with triggers and high-risk situations already. Managing those triggers *is* stress management.

We've also learned about how positive thinking can help us to have healthier core beliefs. Developing healthier core beliefs is another way to manage stress. It's important to remember that we already know how to deal with stress. But knowing how to manage stress is different from practicing what we've learned when we run into stress in our lives.

By planning ahead, we can prepare for when we encounter stress in our lives. As we prepare for release, it can be helpful to outline some positive ways that we have successfully managed stress before. If we make a list of what has worked well for us in the past, we can refer to it when we run into stressful situations. It will remind us of healthy ways to calm down, keep our cool, and maintain a positive attitude.

EXERCISE 7.9   **REFLECTION**

1. What are some healthy things that will help you to feel calm and safe after release?

   _____

   _____

2. What are some healthy things that you plan to do by yourself after release?

   _____

   _____

continued

3. What are some helpful ways you manage stress in your life?

_____

_____

4. How do you plan to manage stressful situations after release?

_____

_____

Managing Mental Health

Some of us have co-occurring disorders and mental health concerns that we will need to manage after release. It is just as important to manage our mental health as it is to manage our physical health. We will need to find a therapist or counselor whom we can meet with regularly after release. We will also want to seek out a recovery support group that understands our condition. If we take medications, we will need to find out where to pick those up after release. We will also want to make sure we take them regularly. A weekly pill organizer may be helpful.

Spiritual Wellness

Think about a power outside of and greater than yourself. It doesn't matter what you call that power. It is selfish to believe we have all the answers in life, and that belief has not served us well. A substance use disorder is a disease that affects our bodies, minds, and spirits. To have a balanced life, we need to focus on *all* of those areas.

Each of us has our own idea of what spirituality means, and we each connect with that idea in our own way. Whatever we believe, admitting that we need more than willpower to keep us abstinent is a huge part of recovery.

This may sound strange, but let's face it—we've believed in many powers greater than ourselves: alcohol and other drugs, money, control, and fame, to name a few. When we ask for help, we realize we aren't alone. We gain hope, and we gain more meaning and purpose in our lives.

EXERCISE 7.10   QUICK REVIEW

Based on what you just read, fill in the blanks to complete these statements.

1. It is just as important to manage our _____ health as it is to manage our physical health.

2. A substance use disorder is a disease that affects our bodies, minds, and _____.

3. When we ask for _____, we realize we aren't alone.

Values and Beliefs

Values are our beliefs, principles, and behaviors—the things we feel good about that help us make wise choices. Consider what values and beliefs are most important to you. Positive values make it possible to live a healthy, rewarding life. When we let go of control and believe in spiritual principles, we can recover in a more balanced way.

If we prioritize our values—figure out which values are most important to us—we can make good choices in life. One way to do this is to learn about other religions and other types of beliefs. We can explore new beliefs by reading about them, watching videos about them, talking with other people who have different beliefs than we do, and more.

We can then think about what we learned and decide what we like and what we don't like—that will help us to understand what our own values and beliefs are. As we learn about others, we may even change our minds about our own beliefs—and that's okay! What is important to us can change over time. Our values and beliefs can give our lives greater purpose, and we can work to make sure that we live our lives in a way that matches what we believe.

EXERCISE 7.11 **REFLECTION**

1. What are some of your personal values and beliefs?

_____

_____

2. What's important to you in life?

_____

_____

3. What sort of person do you want to be? How do you want to be remembered?

_____

_____

4. Share your values and beliefs with your group. What helpful thoughts came out of that discussion?

_____

_____

_____

_____

Our values and beliefs can give our lives greater purpose, and we can work to make sure that we live our lives in a way that matches what we believe.

Community and Culture

We've already talked quite a bit about culture, and our spiritual community is an important part of that. Even if we don't attend religious services, we can still have a spiritual community. Our spiritual community can be any group of people who share our values and beliefs.

Think about the people in your support network. Think about the people you admire. Think about those you reach out to when you need help, and the people you help when they are in need. These are all people who may be part of your spiritual community.

Our spiritual community helps define our spiritual culture. Remember that *culture* refers to a group's beliefs, values, traditions, and customs. Getting more involved in our spiritual community and culture can help our recovery. A spiritual community can be an important support to us after release and can make our reentry much smoother.

EXERCISE 7.12	QUICK REVIEW

Based on what you just read, check *true* or *false* for the statements below.

1. When we let go of control and believe in spiritual principles, we can recover in a more balanced way.

    True _____   False _____

2. We are born with our values and beliefs, and they do not change as we get older.

    True _____   False _____

3. Getting more involved in our spiritual community and culture can help our recovery.

    True _____   False _____

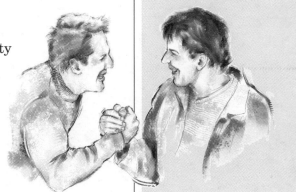

Spiritual Activity

Part of spiritual wellness involves setting aside time to focus on our spirituality. Some of us might already meditate or pray. But there are other activities we can do that boost our spiritual wellness. We can take time to appreciate nature, for example. Or as we just talked about, we can read about other religions and beliefs and discuss what we learned with others.

The point is, to have spiritual wellness, we need to make time for it in our lives. We need to plan activities that involve our values and beliefs, as well as our community and culture. Scheduling and participating in regular spiritual activities that align with our beliefs, traditions, and values after release is a sober and crime-free way to spend time that supports our recovery.

EXERCISE 7.13	REFLECTION

1. List a goal for yourself that supports *physical* wellness after release.

   _____

   _____

   _____

2. List a goal for yourself that supports *emotional* wellness after release.

   _____

   _____

   _____

3. List a goal for yourself that supports *spiritual* wellness after release.

   _____

   _____

   _____

4. How do you plan to achieve these goals?

_____

_____

_____

5. What challenges might you run into?

_____

_____

_____

6. How do you plan to overcome those challenges?

_____

_____

_____

_____

Chapter Summary

In this chapter, we learned about physical wellness and discussed the importance of exercise, sleep, nutrition, preventative care, and sexual health. We also explored emotional wellness and noted the importance of communicating feelings, taking care of ourselves, managing stress, and managing mental health. In addition, we talked about spiritual wellness and discussed the importance of values and beliefs, community and culture, and spiritual activity. Finally, we set goals that will support these areas of our health and wellness after release.

■

Finances

By the end of this chapter, you will be able to	• define what financial wellness looks like after release • explain the basics of budgeting • plan ways to pay off debt after release • plan ways to set aside savings after release

Few of us have been taught how to make good decisions with our money. As a result, many of us may have money troubles. Some of us may have debts we don't know how to repay. On the other hand, some of us are coming out of situations where we've had a lot of money, but we got it illegally. Many people learn about managing money the hard way, but it's never too late to learn how to manage our money. And we *can* learn.

Financial wellness is an important aspect of living a balanced life after release. When we live beyond our means and can't pay our bills, we put ourselves at risk for relapse. Our first priority is to manage money in a way that supports long-term abstinence and recovery. By planning ahead, we can learn more responsible ways to approach our finances after release.

Financial wellness is an important aspect of living a balanced life after release. By planning ahead, we can learn more responsible ways to approach our finances after release.

1. How did you manage money in the past?

_____

_____

2. How would you explain your current state of financial wellness?

_____

_____

3. What are some things that will cost you money after release?

_____

_____

4. How do you hope to improve your financial wellness after release?

_____

_____

Income

Income

The money we make is called our **income.** Our income is different from the money we spend, which is called our **expenses.**

The money we make is called our *income*. We often talk about income in relation to time. All the money that comes in to us during a month is called *monthly income*. All the money that we make over the course of a year is called our *yearly income*. Our income is different from the money we spend, which is called our *expenses*. Learning how to manage our income against our expenses is the basis of financial wellness.

Learning how to manage our income against our expenses is the basis of financial wellness.

Getting a Job

By now, we have discussed the importance of getting a job. We discussed how, in the long run, it is helpful to our recovery to find an honest job doing something that we enjoy. We have already started some planning to help us do that. But it is necessary to find a job that allows us to make enough money to support ourselves. That's why it is helpful to keep track of how much money we make.

When we make money, it is a good idea to put it into the bank. In fact, banks will often pay us a small amount each month just for having an account with them. This is called *interest*. A savings account is really just that—a place where we can save money for later. A savings account usually has a small amount of monthly interest.

A checking account is a little different. With a checking account, the bank manages income and expenses for us. We can deposit money into our account, and we can also write checks or use a debit card to have the bank pay others with the money from our account. Banks do not usually offer interest for a checking account.

Having a bank account allows us to manage our money a little bit easier. Almost everyone has a bank account—people as well as businesses. Some people do keep cash at home, and people do still pay with cash. But most businesses accept debit cards, and it is often easier and safer to use a debit card than it is to carry around cash. After all, if we lose a debit card, the bank will send us a new one. But if we lose cash, we are out of luck.

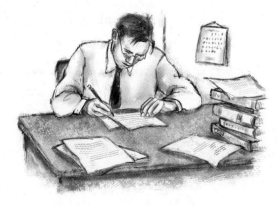

Based on what you just read, fill in the blanks to complete the following statements.

1. Learning how to manage our income against our _____ is the basis of financial wellness.

2. It is necessary to find a job that allows us to make enough money to _____ ourselves.

3. A savings account usually has a small amount of monthly _____ .

4. Having a _____ _____ allows us to manage our money a little bit easier.

Paying Bills

Life would be much better if we only had to deal with income. But we also have to deal with expenses. And there are a lot of expenses in life. For example, we've talked about how we will need to find a place to live after we are released, which means we will probably have to pay monthly rent. *Paying rent* means giving someone else money so we can live in a place that the person owns.

Unfortunately, rent is not the only monthly expense we will have. Some other common expenses include electricity, heating, cable TV, telephone, Internet, and transportation. Most expenses are paid monthly after we receive a bill—a notification telling us how much we owe. It is important to pay our bills on time, because bills that are paid late often have an additional late charge. And late charges can add up quickly. The last thing we want is to end up in a situation where we owe more money than we have—especially if the reason we owe money is because of late fees or overdraft charges!

Expenses

Money we spend is called our **expenses.**

1. What are some concerns you have around income and expenses after release?

_____

_____

_____

_____

2. Where do you plan to keep your income after release?

_____

3. What are some monthly expenses that you know you will have after release?

_____   _____

_____   _____

_____   _____

4. What are some additional expenses that you might have?

_____   _____

_____   _____

_____   _____

Owing a person or a business money is a situation that can create problems for us. We may have faced situations like this in the past that landed us in trouble. But there are things we can do now and after release that will help us to avoid these situations in the future.

Complete a Thinking Report using a situation when we owed more money than we could afford as the event.

> **Thinking Report**

1. **Event** _____

_____

2. **Thoughts** _____

_____

3. **Feelings** _____

_____

4. **Behavior** _____

_____

5. **Core Beliefs** _____

_____

6. **Alternative Thoughts** _____

_____

7. **Alternative Behaviors** _____

_____

Thinking Distortions _____

_____

Thinking Patterns _____

_____

Tactics _____

_____

Budget

One important money-management skill to learn is how to create and stick to a *budget*. A budget is a plan that measures the amount of income against the amount of expenses. Making a budget is one of the most powerful tools we have for keeping our spending under control. We can then use our money for the things that are really important to us.

We might think it makes sense to start our budget by looking at our income. But it is actually better to start by looking at our expenses. After all, once we know what our expenses are, then we can determine how much income we will need.

EXERCISE 8.5	QUICK REVIEW

Based on what you just read, check *true* or *false* for the statements below.

1. Bills that are paid late often have an additional late charge.

    True _____   False _____

2. A budget is a plan that measures the amount of income against the amount of expenses.

    True _____   False _____

3. Making a budget is one of the most powerful tools we have for keeping our spending under control.

    True _____   False _____

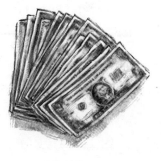

Figuring Out Expenses

To figure out our expenses, we have to look at the different types of expenses we will have. There are three main types of expenses:

- **fixed monthly expenses,** regular expenses that we owe every month

- **periodic expenses,** bills that we only pay once or a few times a year

- **flexible expenses,** things we need or want but can choose how much to spend on

It helps to look at some examples of these expenses so that we can better understand the differences between them. Rent is an example of a fixed monthly expense. We will spend the same amount on rent every month. Good examples of a periodic expense include a new ID card or registration tabs for a car—we don't necessarily pay for them every month, but we do have to pay for them every so often. Examples of flexible expenses include groceries, clothes, or entertainment. It can help if we think about what we *want* versus what we *need*.

Our expenses can all be put into one of those three categories. But to categorize our expenses, we will have to think about all the different types of expenses we have. We may have all three types—fixed, periodic, and flexible—in different areas of our lives.

For example, think about our basic living expenses: we need a place to live, we need to eat, and we need to get to work. So we know that our living expenses will include rent, groceries, and transportation. But we will likely have other living expenses as well. We will need to get our hair cut, for example, and we will also need to pay for laundry (or laundry detergent). If we have children, there are likely even more expenses, but at minimum we may need to pay child support.

Another common expense area is our health. There are many expenses that might fall under this category. For some, it could include fees for a gym membership or teeth cleaning. For others, it could include money for personal hygiene products like toothpaste or over-the-counter medications. Therapy appointments or anger management classes are other possibilities, as are regular donations to support our spiritual community. For those of us with co-occurring disorders, medications may be a necessary expense.

It is also important to consider our social expenses. There are some expenses that would be hard to refuse. For example, it would be hard to turn down requests to help a close family member who needs medical assistance. And we may offer contributions to a recovery support group such as Alcoholics Anonymous, even if it is only a small amount. We also need to set aside a little bit of money for fun, even if we cannot spare much. After all, if we don't set aside some time and money for enjoyment, then we risk burning ourselves out—and that presents a serious risk for relapse.

We have no doubt been thinking about some of the freedom we will gain after release. But reentry does come with expenses, and planning for them now will make them more manageable. Some of those costs are practical. For example, do we have access to any money right away? How will we pay for transportation immediately after release? What can we afford to spend on food when we get out? Other costs will be more strategic. For example, can we afford transportation to a job interview? Can we pay for a career development class? Can we pay for a new uniform when we get a job offer?

"You take a look at the expenses of your life and they do begin to add up. That's why I used to never add them up—too depressing, you know? But the thing is, if you just face it, you can keep it under control. And it's usually not as bad as you think."

— TOM

It can help if we cut down on expenses. Here are some tips for doing that:

- Eat at home when possible, pack a lunch for work, and choose inexpensive restaurants when eating out.

- Cut coupons from newspapers (or print online coupons).

- Look for sales and shop around to make sure to find the best deals.

- Buy in bulk if possible (larger sizes are usually cheaper in the long run).

- Turn down the heat and turn off lights when you're not using them, to save money on energy bills.

- Consider advertising for a roommate to split rent and expenses.

- Ask a landlord if you can do maintenance work in exchange for a rent discount.

- Go without cable television and Internet access.

- Quit or cut down on cigarettes.

- Shop at thrift stores.

- Take public transportation or carpool when possible.

- Buy a good used car rather than a new one; plan efficient routes to save gas.

- Don't pay for warranties—they are often unused or forgotten.

- Use the library for Internet or books.

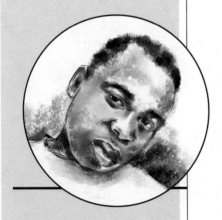

Reentry does come with expenses, and planning for them now will make them more manageable.

Based on what you just read, fill in the blanks to complete the
following statements.

1. We may have all three types of expenses—fixed,
    _____, and flexible—in different areas of our life.

2. We know that our living expenses will include
    _____, groceries, and transportation.

3. For those of us with co-occurring disorders,
    _____ may be a necessary expense.

4. If we don't set aside some time and money for enjoyment,
    then we risk burning ourselves out—and that presents a
    serious risk for _____.

As we can see, we will have expenses in all areas of our lives. It
is important for us to start thinking about what those expenses
will be and to start keeping track of them all. We can sort our
expenses into the three categories: fixed, periodic, and flexible.
That will help us to start a budget, and a budget is a big step
toward financial wellness after release.

EXERCISE 8.7   REFLECTION

1. Think about all the monthly expenses you will have in different
    areas of your life after release. Sort them according to which
    type of expense they are. Use the table on the next page to
    help you.

2. After you have listed all of the expenses you can think of,
    add up the amounts listed in the right column and put the
    total amount of monthly expenses at the bottom.

continued

Monthly Fixed Expenses	Amount

Monthly Periodic Expenses	Amount

Monthly Flexible Expenses	Amount
Total Monthly Amount (If necessary, divide any yearly expenses by twelve to come up with a monthly amount in the rows above.)	

Determining Income

Next, we need to balance our expenses against our income. Our income can come from a variety of sources: hourly or monthly earnings from a job, child support payments, welfare or public assistance, disability payments, financial aid from a school or training program, or money from investments.

Of course, we do not yet have a job, so we can't fill in our income yet. But our total monthly expenses can tell us how much income we will need to pay for all of our expenses. In that sense, determining our monthly expenses will help us determine what type of work we will need to find after release in order to pay our bills. If we have more expenses than income, we will go into debt. And our debt will grow as each month passes, unless we find a way to reduce our expenses or make more income.

When we do get a job, we will want to keep an ongoing record of our expenses and income. This will be our total ongoing budget. Keeping track of our budget will keep us on the road to healthy financial wellness, which will increase our chances of long-term recovery success after release.

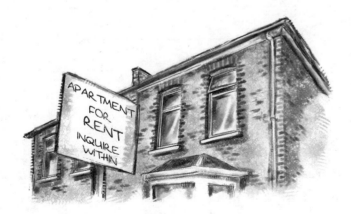

We will have expenses in all areas of our lives.
It is important for us to start thinking about
what those expenses will be and to
start keeping track of them all.

1. Estimate what your monthly income after release will be and list it in the following table. Like you did with expenses earlier, add up the totals in the right column to come up with a total monthly income.

2. Next compare your monthly income against your monthly expenses to see whether you can afford everything on your expense list. If you can't, look at ways you can reduce some of your expenses or consider ways that you might be able to increase your income.

Source of Income	Monthly Amount
Paycheck	
Other	
Other	
Total Monthly Income	

Total Monthly Income	
Total Monthly Expenses	
Difference (Positive + or Negative -)	

Debt

When our expenses are greater than our income, we end up owing a greater amount than we can pay. That's called *debt*. Many of us may have had money troubles in the past when we spent more than we could afford. We may have bought things we really didn't need. Our debt might even have reached the point that we weren't sure how we'd ever be able to repay what we owed.

Being in debt can cause us to feel scared, tense, and worried. It can end up affecting many different areas of our lives and can therefore affect many of our relationships. Paying off debt brings relief and creates opportunities to do things we really want to do. That's why budgeting is so important after release—it can help us pay off any current debt we have, and it can help ensure we avoid more debt in the future.

The first step in dealing with debt is to make a list of our existing debts and the amounts we owe. This list may include

- credit card companies
- student loan companies
- friends or family members who have given us personal loans
- finance companies
- health care organizations
- government agencies (current or back taxes)
- child support
- court fines and fees
- restitution costs

Next, we can decide which debt or debts we should start paying off first. For example, if we are thinking about going back to school, we may want to begin repaying student loans so we will be allowed to register. Sometimes it helps if we pay off smaller debts first, so we feel like we are making progress. If some debts have higher interest rates, we may want to start with those. Consider talking to a banker or a financial planner for advice.

Savings

The goal of a budget is to have more income than expenses. We can use the extra income to pay off our debt. But after we have our debt paid off, we can start to put our extra income into savings. We talked earlier about the difference between a savings account and a checking account. While opening a checking account allows us to make payments with a debit card, it is also a good idea to open a savings account.

We all know that emergencies can happen. And often, emergencies have expenses attached to them. For this reason, it can be helpful to have an emergency fund set aside. That way, when emergencies *do* come up, we can use money from our emergency savings rather than having these unexpected expenses ruin our monthly budget.

It can help to set a goal for how much money we are comfortable putting into an emergency fund. Then we can work toward putting that amount of money aside until we reach our goal. Even if we can only afford to set aside one dollar per paycheck, that's more money for a future emergency than we had before. When we reach our goal, we can pretend that money doesn't exist until an emergency actually happens. That should be the *only* reason we use that money.

Saving money isn't just important for emergencies—it's also important for our future. We won't want to work forever, and we'll need money if we want to retire. Additionally, we'll likely need money for medical expenses as we get older. It helps to start setting aside money now.

Money that is put into savings or investments will earn interest, and the longer it stays there, the more interest it will earn. That means that the earlier we start to set aside money for retirement, the more money we will make. It is also helpful to research where we can get the best interest rate. The higher the interest rate, the more money we will make. Avoid fees whenever possible, since fees just waste the money we worked hard to earn.

The approach to saving money is pretty much the same as it is for paying off debt. We should set aside whatever amount we can, as often as we can. Many employers can actually help us set up retirement funds, and those funds are often tax free. In fact, some employers will even contribute to our retirement. Our banker or a financial planner can offer us savings advice.

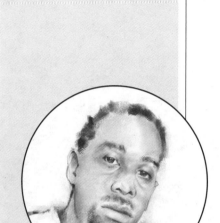

The goal of a budget is to have more income than expenses. We can use the extra income to pay off our debt and begin saving.

Again, it helps to set savings goals. As much as possible, we should try to leave money that we have in savings alone. In fact, some retirement accounts have large fees if we use the money before retirement. We put it in savings for our future, and therefore we should only plan to spend it in the future.

EXERCISE 8.9 **QUICK REVIEW**

Based on what you just read, check *true* or *false* for the following statements.

1. Being in debt is never something to worry about.

    True _____   False _____

2. The first step in dealing with debt is to make a list of our existing debts and the amounts we owe.

    True _____   False _____

3. The goal of a budget is to have more income than expenses.

    True _____   False _____

4. The approach to saving money is pretty much the same as it is for paying off debt.

    True _____   False _____

Credit

The term *credit* refers to how likely someone is to pay back money that is loaned to them. Each person is given a *credit score*. The better our credit score, the more likely we are to be able to get a loan and get lower interest rates. Just like trust between people, no one starts with good credit—we have to earn it.

We earn good credit by paying our bills on time. Cell phone companies, electric companies, and landlords may all report to credit companies on how often we pay our bills. So paying bills on time will help us build credit and keep a good credit score.

Just like trust between people, no one starts with good credit—we have to earn it.

Duplicating this page is illegal. Do not copy this material without written permission from the publisher.

FINANCES • 147

We can also earn credit by paying off credit cards and loans on time, or even early. But to get a loan, we need good credit.

We've all heard of credit cards, but we might not understand how they work. A credit card is like a debit card we get from the bank, but we don't need money in an account to get one. A bank will loan us money and let us use a credit card to pay for things. But they will charge us interest on our debt, so we want to be sure to pay off the debt regularly.

When we pay off our debt on a credit card, our credit score improves. Therefore, it can be good to get a credit card and use it once a month to buy something affordable, such as a haircut. Then, we can make sure we pay our bill every month and we don't risk getting charged interest by the credit card company. This is a good way to build credit.

We have to be careful with credit, however. It can be all too easy to use a credit card on things we want because we don't have to pay for them right away. But if we don't pay for them soon, then we get charged interest on what we owe. And interest rates on credit cards are often very high! In addition, credit card companies often charge late fees if we don't pay the bill on time. Interest and late fees can add up to a lot of debt very quickly, and that makes credit cards risky.

We shouldn't buy *anything* on credit unless we are certain that we can pay it off quickly. Our credit score and history are tracked by large companies. People can request information about our credit score, and they do this when we apply for a loan. It's a good idea to know what our current credit score is, and we can find out by requesting a free copy of our credit report.

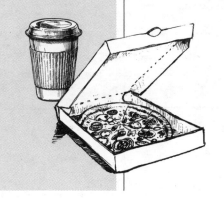

*We have to be careful with credit.
It can be all too easy to use a credit card
on things we want because we
don't have to pay for them right away.*

1. List a goal that will help improve your *financial* wellness after release.

   _____

   _____

2. How do you plan to achieve that goal?

   _____

   _____

   _____

3. What challenges might you run into?

   _____

   _____

   _____

4. How do you plan to overcome those challenges?

   _____

   _____

   _____

Chapter Summary

In this chapter, we learned the definition of *income,* and we discussed how to make money by getting a job and how to responsibly pay bills. We then learned what a budget is and explored a variety of different expenses. We discovered ways to pay off debt, set aside savings, and build credit. Finally, we set a goal to improve our financial wellness after release.

Duplicating this page is illegal. Do not copy this material without written permission from the publisher.

FINANCES • **149**

Mapping
Your Release

By the end of this chapter, you will be able to	• develop goals for the first day after release
	• develop goals for the first week after release
	• develop long-term goals for after release

We've done a lot of planning in this workbook for our lives after release. We've set goals around living under supervision, a healthy recovery environment, a healthy support network, occupational success, healthy free time, health and wellness, and finances. That's a lot of work, and we deserve credit for planning a healthy future for ourselves after release.

But our work isn't done. In fact, in some ways our work is just beginning. Setting recovery goals is one thing, but achieving them is another. We've made some important changes to our lives, and those changes have paved a new path forward for us.

Reentry will be a transition from the structured environment we find ourselves in now to one where we have a lot more freedom. But as Eleanor Roosevelt once famously said, "With freedom comes great responsibility." As we prepare for release, we can use what we've learned to put our goals into action. We're ready to show ourselves and the rest of the world that the path we're following now is the path to successful recovery.

"With freedom comes great responsibility."

—ELEANOR ROOSEVELT

Planning Your First Day

Exploring a new place is much easier when we have a map. But first someone needs to create that map. We have everything we need to create a map for our new life after release, and we know that we're the best person for the job.

The first step is always the hardest, and our first few days after release are our first steps toward long-term recovery. We can look at the goals we've created in this workbook and use them to create a plan for after release.

EXERCISE **9.1**	**REFLECTION**

Take a look at the goals you set at the end of each chapter in this workbook. Then use them to create a list of goals for your first day after release.

1. List a goal related to living under supervision during your first day after release.

   _____

   _____

   Explain how you plan to achieve your goal.

   _____

   _____

2. List a goal related to finding a healthy recovery environment during your first day after release.

   _____

   _____

   Explain how you plan to achieve your goal.

   _____

   _____

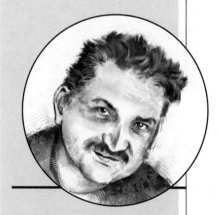

Relapse prevention and recovery support will be most critical in the days just after our release.

3. List a goal related to finding a healthy support network during your first day after release.

_____

_____

Explain how you plan to achieve your goal.

_____

_____

4. List an occupational goal during your first day after release.

_____

_____

Explain how you plan to achieve your goal.

_____

_____

5. List a goal related to healthy ways to spend free time during your first day after release.

_____

_____

Explain how you plan to achieve your goal.

_____

_____

6. List a goal related to health and wellness during your first day after release.

_____

_____

continued

We've made some important changes to our lives, and those changes have paved a new path forward for us.

Explain how you plan to achieve your goal.

_____

_____

7. List a goal related to healthy finances during your first day after release.

_____

_____

Explain how you plan to achieve your goal.

_____

_____

8. Describe in detail what you plan to do on your first day. It may be helpful to plan something for every hour of the day.

_____

_____

_____

_____

_____

_____

_____

_____

_____

9. Share your plan for your first day with your group. What helpful thoughts came out of that discussion?

_____

_____

Planning Your First Week

We will likely find our first week a little bit easier than our first day, but it will still be helpful to make a plan for the week. Use the goals you listed for your first day after release to help you create additional goals for your first week after release.

EXERCISE 9.2	REFLECTION

1. List a goal related to living under supervision during your first week after release.

   _____

   _____

   Explain how you plan to achieve your goal.

   _____

   _____

2. List a goal related to finding a healthy recovery environment during your first week after release.

   _____

   _____

   Explain how you plan to achieve your goal.

   _____

   _____

3. List a goal related to finding a healthy support network during your first week after release.

   _____

   _____

   Explain how you plan to achieve your goal.

   _____

   _____

continued

Duplicating this page is illegal. Do not copy this material without written permission from the publisher.

MAPPING YOUR RELEASE • 155

4. List an occupational goal during your first week after release.

_____

_____

Explain how you plan to achieve your goal.

_____

_____

5. List a goal related to healthy ways to spend free time during your first week after release.

_____

_____

Explain how you plan to achieve your goal.

_____

_____

6. List a goal related to health and wellness during your first week after release.

_____

_____

Explain how you plan to achieve your goal.

_____

_____

7. List a goal related to healthy finances during your first week after release.

_____

_____

Explain how you plan to achieve your goal.

_____

_____

8. Describe a general schedule for each day of your first week after release.

_____

_____

_____

_____

9. Share your plan for your first week with your group. What helpful thoughts came out of that discussion?

_____

_____

Long-Term Planning

Now that we've set goals for the first day and the first week after release, it's time to plan for the long term. Use the recovery goals you set for the first day after release and the first week after release to set long-term recovery goals.

| EXERCISE 9.3 | REFLECTION |

1. List a long-term goal related to living under supervision.

_____

_____

Explain how you plan to achieve your goal.

_____

_____

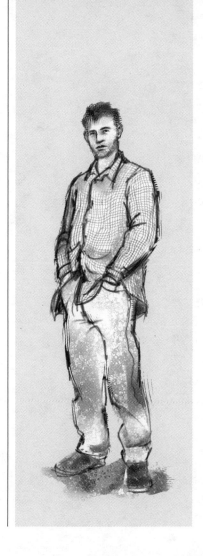

continued

2. List a long-term goal related to finding a healthy recovery environment.

_____

_____

Explain how you plan to achieve your goal.

_____

_____

3. List a long-term goal related to finding a healthy support network.

_____

_____

Explain how you plan to achieve your goal.

_____

_____

4. List a long-term occupational goal.

_____

_____

Explain how you plan to achieve your goal.

_____

_____

5. List a long-term goal related to healthy ways to spend free time.

_____

_____

Explain how you plan to achieve your goal.

_____

_____

6. List a long-term goal related to health and wellness.

_____

_____

Explain how you plan to achieve your goal.

_____

_____

7. List a long-term goal related to healthy finances.

_____

_____

Explain how you plan to achieve your goal.

_____

_____

8. Describe how you can use all your long-term recovery goals in a long-term recovery plan.

_____

_____

_____

9. Share your long-term recovery goals with your group. What helpful thoughts came out of that discussion?

_____

_____

Chapter Summary

We're about to be released. Here are some important points to remember as we begin our new lives:

- **Our recovery is our number one priority.** Every decision we make and every action we take must support our abstinence.

- **We need to be flexible.** We have to remember that things don't always go according to plan and that we always have options. We need to be flexible in how we react.

- **We need to have goals.** Our goals should be SMART goals. It's okay to think big. Over time, we can make a lot of progress.

- **Stress and frustration will happen.** This doesn't mean we're doing something wrong. It means we're trying and we're growing. Stress and frustration happen to everybody.

Remember, it's good to start each day with a schedule. And it's helpful to follow this schedule as closely as we can. But we shouldn't let this schedule be *too* rigid. If we aren't able to follow our schedule exactly as planned, that's okay. It's also good practice to try and avoid planning several important events in a row. Again, it helps to be flexible.

Attitude Is Important

When something goes wrong, the outcome is never as bad as we might fear. *Remember, there are always options.* Job interviews can be rescheduled. There are ways to make up material covered in missed classes. We need to relax and take it in stride. If we're always on edge, convinced that one mistake will become a crisis, we risk a setback. And we may put ourselves at risk for relapse.

When something goes wrong, the outcome is never as bad as we might fear. Remember, there are always options.

Congratulations! By doing the work in this workbook, you've accomplished something big. Take this workbook with you once you're released—it's your map for your new life as an abstinent person. By following your plans in this workbook, your chances of long-term recovery are greatly improved.

You've got a chance to approach life from a whole new angle. You've prepared yourself. You've put in the work that shows you're committed to success. If you put in the same effort once you're released, one day others will see you and say, "There's someone who made it. That person proves it's possible."

Notes

Chapter 3

1. The Wellness Wheel is adapted from the Eight Dimensions of Wellness graphic in *Creating a Healthier Life: A Step-by-Step Guide to Wellness,* SMA16-4958 (Rockville, MD: Substance Abuse and Mental Health Services Administration, 2016), which in turn is adapted from Margaret Swarbrick, "A Wellness Approach," *Psychiatric Rehabilitation Journal* 29, no. 4 (2006): 311–14.

Chapter 7

1. National Institutes of Health, "The Importance of Sleep," *NIH Medline Plus* 7, no. 2 (Summer 2012): 17, https://medlineplus.gov/magazine/issues/summer12/articles/summer12pg17.html.

2. U.S. Department of Health and Human Services, "Get Enough Sleep," https://healthfinder.gov/HealthTopics/Category/everyday-healthy-living/mental-health-and-relationship/get-enough-sleep#the-basics_3.

Thinking Report

1. **Event** _____
   _____

2. **Thoughts** _____
   _____

3. **Feelings** _____
   _____

4. **Behavior** _____
   _____

5. **Core Beliefs** _____
   _____

6. **Alternative Thoughts** _____
   _____

7. **Alternative Behaviors** _____
   _____

Thinking Distortions _____
_____

Thinking Patterns _____
_____

Tactics _____
_____

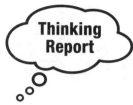

Thinking Report

1. Event _____

_____

2. Thoughts _____

_____

3. Feelings _____

_____

4. Behavior _____

_____

5. Core Beliefs _____

_____

6. Alternative Thoughts _____

_____

7. Alternative Behaviors _____

_____

Thinking Distortions _____

_____

Thinking Patterns _____

_____

Tactics _____

_____

My Notes

My Notes

My Notes

About Hazelden Publishing

As part of the Hazelden Betty Ford Foundation, Hazelden Publishing offers both cutting-edge educational resources and inspirational books. Our print and digital works help guide individuals in treatment and recovery, and their loved ones. Professionals who work to prevent and treat addiction also turn to Hazelden Publishing for evidence-based curricula, digital content solutions, and videos for use in schools, treatment programs, correctional programs, and electronic health records systems. We also offer training for implementation of our curricula.

Through published and digital works, Hazelden Publishing extends the reach of healing and hope to individuals, families, and communities affected by addiction and related issues.

For more information about Hazelden publications,
please call **800-328-9000**
or visit us online at **hazelden.org/bookstore**.